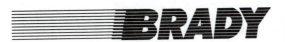

Burnout to Balance:

EMS STRESS

JUDI LIGHT HOPSON
**Hopson/Hopson/Hagen Education Group,
Johnson City, Tennessee**

EMMA H. HOPSON, R.N.
**Hopson/Hopson/Hagen Education Group,
Johnson City, Tennessee**

JEFF T. DYAR, EMT-P
**EMS Program Chair,
National Fire Academy,
Emmitsburg, Maryland**

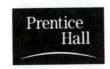

Prentice
Hall

Upper Saddle River, NJ 07458

Library of Congress Cataloging-in-Publication Data

Publisher: Julie Alexander
Aquisitions Editors: Judy Streger and Katrin
  Beacom
Director of Manufacturing and Production: Bruce
  Johnson
Managing Production Editor: Patrick Walsh
Production Editor: Danielle Newhouse
Art Director: Marianne Frasco
Manufacturing Manager: Ilene Sanford
Marketing Manager: Tiffany Price
Marketing Coordinator: Cindy Frederick
Editorial Assistant: Jeanne Molenaar
Cover Designer: Bruce Kenselaar
Cover Image: S. Stephanie Lipson
Interior Designer: Danielle Newhouse
Composition: Rainbow Graphics, LLC
Printing and Binding: RR Donnelley & Sons
  Company

This book is dedicated to all emergency responders and their families and to Doug Fiske, editor of the former Emergency *magazine.*

Doug Fiske's constant praise of our writing and research throughout the years is deeply appreciated. His willingness to publish articles relating to stress management and self-help issues for emergency responders was the foundation for this book.

PRENTICE HALL INTERNATIONAL (UK) LIMITED, London
PRENTICE-HALL OF AUSTRALIA PTY. LIMITED, Sydney
PRENTICE-HALL CANADA, INC., Toronto
PRENTICE-HALL HISPANOAMERICANA, S.A., Mexico
PRENTICE-HALL OF INDIA PRIVATE LIMITED, New Delhi
PRENTICE-HALL OF JAPAN, INC., Tokyo
PRENTICE-HALL SINGAPORE PTE. LTD
EDITORA PRENTICE-HALL DO BRASIL, LTDA., Rio de Janeiro

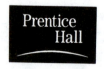

10 9 8 7 6 5 4 3 2 1
ISBN 0-13-007806-9

CONTENTS

PREFACE

Over the past several years, we have collectively spent over 20,000 hours researching stress management issues for EMS personnel, public safety officers, and health-care employees. In researching those issues, we have learned how resourceful an individual must be in order to manage the pressures of daily life. It takes specific coping skills every step of the way to attain success in one's work life and personal life. This book reveals many of those skills and how to apply them.

We have talked with EMTs and paramedics from every state and several Canadian provinces. Law enforcement officers and firefighters who are cross-trained in EMS have shared their perspectives as well. Chaplains, doctors, nurses, mental health professionals, social workers, hospital administrators, EMS administrators, and experts on stress management have also assisted us by sharing their philosophies and experiences.

Meeting those of you who have so generously revealed your private stress issues, hopes, dreams, fears, and frustrations has been an interesting journey. For these very personal conversations, we owe you a huge debt. Both responders and administrators have revealed their deepest pain and their most positive experiences. Each, *without exception,* has expressed the need for more education concerning stress management in the EMS field. Our deepest desire is that our book will meet part of that need.

This book is a reader-friendly guide that we perceive as both an educational resource and a career management tool. We believe that readers will refer to it for many years to come. Our approach is to address both work and personal–family issues because life must be managed as a whole. It is virtually impossible to neatly compartmentalize one's areas of responsibilities. We believe that it is easier to make wiser choices on a daily basis if these areas of responsibility can be perceived as flowing together.

One of our goals was to compile the best techniques for managing stress in a text that is enjoyable to read. We feel that the personal case studies related herein add richness and depth to the text. In addition, firsthand accounts often make serious subjects easier to digest. These personal stories enhance and give clarity to the educational concepts we want to share. Note that all names have been changed to protect privacy.

This book offers much information about how individuals can find and give emotional support, develop healthier relationships, and deal with politics in the workplace. It also emphasizes self-nurturing and career planning. Managing all of the issues of EMS work-related stress is a monumental challenge, especially for those who work in busy urban areas or rural areas with few resources. Some responders are facing "burnout" whereas others are confronted with boredom—often referred to as "rustout"—because of infrequent calls or other problems within a work setting. We address both issues in this text.

This book offers advice to steer both newcomers and veterans to clear methods of stress management. Above all, our desire is to offer concrete tips for how stress reduction can be brought under one's control *without a great deal of dependence on others.* We also want to demonstrate that it is the smallest of control measures that can begin to turn the tide of stress. The methods of stress management we share show readers that making a series of minor changes in several areas is the way to begin. We not only help to identify certain control buttons but also share with readers how to activate them. By consistently taking steps for positive change, one can find more inner harmony and a sense of life satisfaction.

We have organized the chapters of the book so that they can be read out of sequence, if the reader so desires. This book is a practical guide interwoven with self-help techniques for both supervisory and nonsupervisory personnel. We intend that each faction can reflect on the issues and experiences of the other. For example, by having a fuller understanding of the stress issues of personnel under one's supervision, it is easier to encourage teamwork and work to reduce tension among individuals. Conversely, when responders comprehend more about the stress issues of their supervisors, they gain a better understanding of how to carry out their roles in an appropriate way.

We hope that readers will refer to this book often and actively implement many of the ideas for positive change. But above all, we envision that this book will assist individuals in inventing stress management techniques of their own for specific situations. Once basic concepts of stress management are understood, it should become easier for individuals to develop personal coping strategies.

Our work in writing and researching this book has been a personal privilege. This book was written for those actively involved in or preparing to become involved in the EMS field. However, it is also our hope that the families and friends of responders might study it also. Perhaps some of the ideas will help them learn more about assisting responders in building happy, healthy lives. Our wish is that these stress management techniques will enhance the quality of life for those who sacrifice so much for the well-being of our society.

Judi Light Hopson
Emma H. Hopson
Jeff T. Dyar

ACKNOWLEDGMENTS

We would like to thank the individuals who made specific contributions to the completion of this book: Troy Doman and S. Stephanie Lipson for their illustrations; Karen Cassell for her research; Shanna Light, Jean Hobson, and Toumonava Nelson for their editing; Doug Harris for computer tech support; and Marcie Roth for typing the manuscript.

All of the following individuals also offered their help in a variety of ways: Michael Cassell, Mary Ellen Wilkin, Dr. Carla Warner.

A special thank-you to our family and friends. The following people gave either hands-on help with the book or emotional support throughout the project: James Hopson, Mark Hopson, Lauren Hopson, Beth and Carl Light, Liz and Ray Hughes, Priscilla Harris, Sherri Backers, Randall and Amy Light, Chris Light, Shelby McCoy Light, Carson Light, Florence Baker.

We'd also like to thank the following reviewers for their suggestions and feedback:

Brenda Beasley, RN, BS, EMT-P
EMS Program Director
Calhoun College
Decatur, AL

Donald Bloom
Vice President
Penn Care
Niles, OH

Sandra (Sam) Bradley, MICP
Field Training Coordinator
American Medical Response
Los Medanos College
Livermore, CA

Gary Davis
EMS Coordinator
Chief
Oklahoma City Fire Department
Oklahoma City, OK

T.J. Feldman, MA, EMT-B
Avon, CT

J. Scott Hartley, EMS-I, NREMT-P
A.L.S. Affiliates
Omaha, NE

Arthur Hsieh, BS, NREMT-P
San Francisco Fire Department
EMS Division
San Francisco, CA

Joe "Kuby" Kubitschek, MICT, CCEMT-P
Russell Regional Hospital
Russell, KS

Tim Murphy, NREMT-P
EMS Educational Coordinator
Carl Sandburg College
Galesburg, IL

Stephen J. Nardozzi
Chairperson, Department of Prehospital EMS
Westchester Community College
Valhalla, NY

Michael J. O'Brien
St. Vincent Hospital
Indianapolis, IN

Lt. Tim Peebles
EMS Instructor
Hall County Fire Services
Gainesville, GA

John S. Senft
Deputy Chief
Department of Fire/Rescue Services
City of York
York, PA

Patricia Stafford, EMT-P
Director of Education
Gateway Ambulance
St. Louis Community College
St. Louis, MO

Gail A. Stewart
Coordinator, EMS Programs
Santa Fe Community College
Gainesville, FL

Michael Sturgill, NREMT-P
Education and Training Coordinator
American Medical Response—South Mississippi
Gulfport, MS

Barbara Zeglin, BA, EMT-B, NREMT-B
Lehigh Community College
Dallas, PA

ABOUT THE AUTHORS

Judi Light Hopson is an author and journalist who specializes in psychology topics. For over 25 years, she has written for numerous magazines including *Essence, Columbia, Home Life, Catholic Digest, Christian Single, Living with Children, Mature Living, St. Anthony Messenger, Signs of the Times,* and *Equal Opportunity.*

She was a contributing writer and columnist for the former *Emergency* magazine for five years. Her topics for the magazine focused on stress management and emotional well-being.

Judi's feature articles have appeared in major newspapers such as the *San Francisco Chronicle,* the *Chicago Tribune,* the *Christian Science Monitor,* and the *Miami Herald.* Her work has been syndicated worldwide by the Christian Science Monitor Radio News Service, United Feature Syndicate, and Universal Press Syndicate.

She presently co-authors the national newpaper column *Person-to-Person* with Emma H. Hopson, R.N., and Ted Hagen, Ph.D. The column, which offers advice on work and family issues, is distributed to more than 300 newspapers by Knight-Ridder/Tribune Information Services, Washington, D.C.

Judi lives with her husband James near the Johnson City, Tennessee, area.

Emma H. Hopson, R.N., is a writer who has worked in the medical field for over 20 years. She has held administrative positions, including manager of a 32-bed ICU and clinical manager of the ER, at the Johnson City Medical Center in Tennessee.

Her articles have appeared in such magazines as *Emergency, Columbia,* and *St. Anthony Messenger.* She also co-authors the national newspaper column *Person-to-Person* with Judi Light Hopson and Ted Hagen, Ph.D., a psychologist.

Emma teaches seminars on career development for health care professionals and speaks regularly on self-help psychology topics.

Currently, she is the director of nursing for a long-term care facility. She resides with her husband of 20 years and their daughter in upper east Tennessee.

Jeff Dyar is EMS program chair at the National Fire Academy in Emmitsburg, Maryland. His lifelong career in EMS began 30 years ago as a volunteer on a small-town ambulance service. He also served as a U.S. Army Medic. Jeff is an alumnus paramedic of Swedish Medical Center, Denver, Colorado. His experience includes service in public, third service, and private ALS-EMS organizations and as a career firefighter. Jeff has held academic posts at the university level and developed and directed paramedic-level training programs.

Jeff was recognized at a White House presidential ceremony for his contributions to the Reinvention of Government program. He is also a recipient of the James O. Page Lifetime Achievement Award from the International Association of Fire Chiefs for national leadership in EMS and the fire service.

As an author, his writing and editing contributions include books, journals, college-level EMS management courses, and advisory positions for several media companies.

Jeff is the CEO of the Far View Group (www.farviewgroup.com) and is a featured presenter and educator-facilitator at national EMS and fire service conferences. His wife and two sons support him in these interests and efforts.

CHAPTER ONE

ESCAPING OVERLOAD

Do you feel pulled in so many directions that you worry you will snap like a rubber band? Managing your job stress and personal life has become too complicated. All of the demands placed upon you have you feeling as if you are on a runaway train. You would like to slow down the madness. But you can't just throw on the brakes. Your work would suffer. Your life might crash. So how can you slow down the train, find more balance, and regain control?

Emergency Medical Services educators are always emphasizing the importance of good self-care. You already comprehend what constitutes a healthy diet. You know how to exercise. You have also memorized lots of tips on how emergency responders can cope. But it's not enough. The pressures of too much work, too few rewards, and an overall depressed feeling have you singing the burnout blues.

Whether you're fed up a little or a lot, you can find your way out of the maze of madness. The advice in this book will help you regain control of your work life and home life. We offer you the tools for taking very small, manageable steps out of the craziness. We also show you that *taking this control can be an enjoyable experience.*

BUILDING YOUR OWN BRIDGES

Whether you are an EMT who is burning out after 4 years, or an EMS manager who has supervised 75 people for 15 years, you need your own tailor-made plan for improving your situation. We show you how to be the architect in designing this plan. If you're new in EMS, you will learn how to cope with stress before you approach the burnout state.

Every single emergency responder or supervisor has his or her own unique set of personal stress factors. What's stressful to one individual might not bother an-

1

other. What gets one person down might seem insignificant to someone else. The bottom line is that you're entitled to "own" your feelings—just as they are. By getting in touch with what makes you happy or sad, you can start constructing bridges to where you want to go.

Although no one typically "gets it all" in this life, you can still get your healthy share of a life that's rewarding, both personally and professionally. You can find enough balance to feel good about yourself and what you do. EMS is a special field. The learning opportunities are endless. There's almost nothing you cannot do in connection with this line of work. For example, you can speak, teach, write, learn budgets, do mechanical work, and help your community. You can also use computer skills, invent equipment to help save lives, utilize public relations skills, travel to conferences, meet interesting people, work with public officials, and, most of all, learn transferable skills for other professions, related or unrelated to EMS.

All of these possibilities might not sound appealing at the moment. In fact, perhaps you would prefer to run off to a mountain cabin for a month. If it weren't for that stack of unpaid bills on your kitchen counter, you might seriously consider it. You might feel so tired, so unmotivated at times, that you can't think straight. You need advice on stress that you can implement easily without causing yourself further stress.

This book will guide you from *burnout to balance* in ways that work. Most importantly, the majority of these steps are ones you can take by yourself—without counting too much on other people to change. There's an old adage that says: "Nothing changes. We change." But therein lies the key to reducing stress in your life: *When you are self-directed, you have more control.*

Getting off overload will be something you must do your way. You are the best expert on yourself and your life. You know what will work for you. We show you that you have more options than you might think.

SLOWING DOWN THE TRAIN

As you're speeding along on the runaway train of stress, think about the boxcars as areas of responsibility that you are hauling. By using this analogy of boxcars, you can envision the separate loads you're carrying in your daily routine such as family, work, finances, and community obligations. With yourself as the engine of this train, picture how tired you're getting chugging along with boxcars that are too full.

If you could slow your train down and find time to think, you might figure ways to lighten your load. Could you ditch freight that you don't need? Could you drop a boxcar entirely? If you could manage to balance your load, you could then speed back up. The benefits of slowing down to think and make changes will pay off in the long run. You can go farther on your career track when your train is lighter and more manageable. Start with five minutes a day, if that's all you have. Spend this time reflecting on how to gain control over your different areas of responsibility.

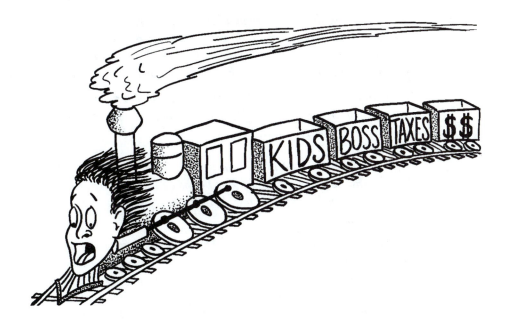

Let's get started . . .

As you think about what is troubling you—a boss who's demanding too much, employees who are getting on your nerves, or a marriage that needs work—take control by resolving to change at least one minor thing this week.

1. Make a list of your major stress areas.
2. Identify one small change in each area that might help.
3. Implement a change to see if it helps. If it does not, try another one until something "clicks."
4. Resolve to make small changes consistently, until you feel more in control in all areas.

Here are examples of how two people regained a sense of control over problems by using this method:

Dan, an EMT whose wife Diana was fed up with their erratic schedules, felt he was headed for divorce court. "We had no quality time together," says Dan. "We were losing each other and we both knew it." Dan told his wife, "Let's try to calm things down in our lives so that our time together is not always centered on problems."

Dan and Diana decided to spend 15 minutes just embracing each other every time they were together. They sat on the couch or lay quietly in bed together. "We didn't talk or discuss anything," Dan emphasizes. "We used the power of touch to connect. We told our kids they could sit or lie close, but they had to be quiet."

He continues, "After we got the hang of holding each other, we worked on listening to each other. Next, we bought some tapes on relationships. It took time, but we got our marriage on track."

Angie, a supervisor of 12 EMTs and paramedics in an urban EMS station in the Southeast, was stressed out because her house was cluttered. After a grueling shift at work, she hated facing toys, laundry, newspapers, and junk all over her three-bedroom home.

"I vowed to take control," says Angie. "Every week I bought one tool for getting organized. For example, the first week I spent ten dollars on hooks for hanging things in the children's rooms. The next week, I bought five cheap laundry baskets for sorting toys and junk. I just kept at it until I got the house under control. It was a slow process, but I told myself, 'Every week I'll do something positive.' "

Getting your life off overload calls for having a plan that is simple. When you're really stressed, the last thing you need is a plan that is too tough to implement. Although your steps should be easy in the beginning, you can gradually move to bigger and bolder steps. But initially, *think baby steps, not quantum leaps,* in reducing the pressure.

Here are some crucial steps for lowering stress at work:

- **When you feel overwhelmed, force yourself to plan.** Tension eases somewhat when you find a control button—even a tiny one. Look at all of your options in a situation. If none of those options look acceptable, try to create one by asking "How would I advise someone else to handle this?"
- **Start using more positive language.** Language has the power to shape our lives. Speaking more positively will help anyone under stress feel more in control. By saying "I'm sure I can find a way to cope," you're giving yourself hope and a positive sense of direction. If possible, avoid individuals who speak too negatively.
- **Remind yourself of all the things you are doing right.** By patting yourself on the back and *focusing on what's going well,* you can energize yourself. *Focusing on the negative will drain you faster than anything.*
- **Clearly define your emotional limit with each patient, coworker, employee, and business associate.** State to each individual: "Here's what I can do," or "Here's what I can accomplish." Give enough to feel

good about yourself, but decide where to draw the line in terms of mental energy expended.

Reminder

When you define your limits with others, *be as nice as you can, but be as specific as you can concerning what you can and cannot do.*

For instance, if you have a friend who's always dumping personal problems on you, simply say: "I can listen to you for ten minutes, but I'm too busy to go beyond that. Please understand that I'm overloaded today myself."

If this is difficult for you to say, try practicing the words with a friend or family member.

More about defining limits . . .

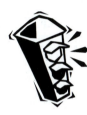 So how can you better handle stress and define your limits if a bad scene is haunting you? Try to process a scene in a way that helps you obtain "closure"—a mental shelf to put it on. Although this is too simplistic for truly intense calls, which may require critical incident stress debriefing or personal counseling, there are ways to bring closure to many incidents. For example, you should try to identify the hard parts of each emergency call and then *frame the experiences in ways that spell hope, not despair.*

Here are some tips for thinking about stressful calls in which you were involved:

- **Whenever possible, try to interpret trying experiences in ways that are positive.** Be grateful that you could help in any way. A positive approach will help to reinforce your self-esteem, which is a big factor in avoiding burnout.

- **Process your work through your mind in ways that help you work toward closure.** Too many loose ends, unanswered questions, and inner conflict about errors on the job will disempower you—accelerating stress.

- **Track down information.** If you want to know what became of a particular person at a scene, or if you feel uneasy about something at a scene, try to get the information you need to ease your mind. Even if a tiny, seemingly insignificant detail is bothering you, define the detail, talk about it, and then find a mental shelf to put it on.

Backing away from anxiety over a difficult conversation or a difficult scene is harder for some individuals. For example, your work role can affect how you cope with issues. If you're in a management position, you can't turn off problems by saying "I don't have time to talk" or "I feel good about how I handled myself on that call." Your worries are more complex.

Let's say that you run a private ambulance company where employees are quarreling and the budget is strained. On top of these pressures, you have a spouse who feels neglected and you don't have time to visit the dentist. Just thinking about your problems gives you a splitting headache.

An example of how to begin acquiring balance, implementing the one-step tactic to get things moving in the right direction is shown in Table 1.1:

TABLE 1.1

PROBLEM	SMALL CHANGE TO TRY
Two EMTs are arguing almost daily. They're causing tension in the troops, which is affecting morale. A face-to-face meeting with management hasn't worked.	Require them to put their grievances against each other in writing—complete with suggestions on improving work strategies. Make them think logically about their pettiness.
Money is running out for equipment and supplies. Worrying over the budget has you tossing in your sleep. The owner of the company has fully delegated budget problems to you.	With the owner's permission, phone an accountant who works with budgets similar to yours (for example, the police department or another private EMS service comparable to yours). Ask this person to take a look at your books and offer suggestions.
Your spouse wants more quality time with you. You're too tired to give it.	Make one-minute "I miss you" calls twice daily.
You need to visit the dentist, but finding the time looks impossible for weeks.	Postpone a meeting for personnel that can wait. Or, delegate your role in the meeting to a trusted subordinate.

ATTITUDE GOES A LONG WAY

Whether you're still riding the adrenaline high of your first years in EMS, or you're so burned out that a hospital stay sounds like a vacation, you can manage stress better if you program your brain properly. Your brain is your personal computer in every sense. Positive self-messages, or self-talk, will put you ahead in conserving your mental energy.

Below are some coping tools for your tool kit. Try repeating statements such as these to yourself four or five times when stress is clouding your day.

I'll picture how an efficient person would do my job.

Tell yourself that you can model your performance after someone who could step into your shoes and do an excellent job. What attitude would this person have? What kinds of methods would he or she use in communicating better with coworkers? How would your role model handle difficult patients?

I'll remind myself of my strong points.

It's important to believe in yourself when the going gets tough. It's easier to bring out the best in yourself, and do work you are proud of, if you focus on your strengths. It's okay to *feed your ego by continually looking at your attributes.* If you believe in yourself, others will also.

I'll learn to manage frustration.

No one ever accomplished great things in any profession without learning to handle great amounts of frustration. *A job with few frustrations probably has few rewards.* Remind yourself that you can learn to confront frustration, step around it, and keep going. This attitude is crucial for conserving mental energy.

I'll define my stumbling block and find my way around it.

Tell yourself you'll *identify what is hindering real progress* in any situation. The stumbling block can be indecisiveness or fear of facing the truth about a scenario. Lack of self-honesty about your need for more education, new skills, or help from your boss could keep you stuck in a stressful situation. When identifying a stumbling block, ask yourself, "Do I need to change something about myself?"

Being honest about things that are out of your control saves emotional energy.

Indecisiveness and worry give your brain unclear signals, which hinder intelligent action. Always be clear with yourself about what your role in EMS entails. Don't require something of yourself that is impossible for you to perform or know.

What you say when you talk to yourself is probably the main key to keeping all stress under control. But the statements you use must be believable and as specific as possible. They should not obscure good judgment nor keep the truth hidden.

For example, there are times when you should tell yourself, "I'm not perfect and I will make mistakes. I don't demand perfection from myself, but I'm determined to improve my skills. I will learn something from every error." Try using positive self-communication to assess a situation honestly, and then *coach yourself with messages that bring out the best in you.*

Self-coaching can also help you wind down emotionally after a killer day. By saying "I want to stay home tonight and relax, and that's exactly what I'm going to do," your mind is signaled that rest is definitely forthcoming. You're talking to yourself in an emotionally supportive way.

SLEEP . . . THE GREATEST STRESSBUSTER

When you are under enormous stress, it is wise to use many strategies to reduce stress. However, a main key to mental well-being is, and always will be, sleep. The importance of getting sufficient sleep can't be overemphasized. However, the long hours, difficult schedules, and emotional pressures of EMS life make getting *enough* sleep hard to acquire. But you can focus on enhancing the *quality* of your sleep.

> *An EMT we'll call Jack found himself so stressed that he hadn't slept two hours straight in a month. He was living and working in a mental fog. "I was popping caffeine pills when I needed to be alert," Jack confesses. "But when it was time to sleep, I couldn't. The caffeine certainly didn't help. However, the underlying causes of my problems were emotional."*
>
> *Jack had gone through a difficult divorce, plus he'd had to declare bankruptcy. He was working one full-time and one part-time job at two different EMS stations. "During this time, my dad had a near-fatal heart attack," Jack explains. "Then two weeks later, my son was diagnosed with a serious illness."*
>
> *No wonder Jack couldn't sleep. It's a miracle he could function at all. Surprisingly, he did manage to get back on track without taking a lot of medication or losing a lot of work. "Under a doctor's care, I stayed off work for ten days to get my sleep back in rhythm," he points out. "I took prescribed sleeping pills. I also*

got into private counseling for four months. The counseling helped. But I did two things to make sleep more comfortable.

"Though I couldn't afford it, I bought myself an expensive mattress," continues Jack. "Don't laugh. Three solid hours of sleep on a good mattress beats six hours of tossing around on a lumpy one. Next, I got a mattress factory to donate thirty top-of-the-line mattresses to our EMS station. Our old mattresses were ready for the garbage."

These tips for sleeping better might help you improve your situation:

- **Remember that you can fall asleep easier if you don't eat a lot of protein before bedtime, especially beef or pork.** Protein is metabolized in a way that triggers alertness in the brain. Consume protein early in the day and stick with mostly carbohydrates—cereal, vegetables, pasta— during the four hours before bedtime.

- **It is much easier to fall asleep in a very dark room.** Invest in room-darkening shades. It can be very hard to fall asleep in the daytime in a room without shades. Even if you feel sleepy, it can be almost impossible to do anything but catnap. Your eyelids are thin enough to allow a small amount of light to filter through.

- **Don't have a beer or mixed drink before bedtime.** Alcohol will make you sleepy at first. But, as a stimulant, it will cause you to wake up about an hour after falling asleep. It will actually interrupt sleep rhythms much like caffeine does. Because a complete sleep "cycle" is ninety minutes—and you need at least four cycles per sleep period— waking up causes you to start one of your sleep cycles over. This can be exhausting.

- **It's easier to sleep if you're having pleasant thoughts.** Do this by creating a "safe place" in your mind to visit before falling asleep. Use your imagination to picture yourself lying on a beach or sleeping out in nature at your favorite camping spot. Negative thoughts, worries, or thinking about a bad call will stimulate your body to wake up.

- **Having a bedtime ritual helps you fall asleep faster.** A cup of hot herbal tea or reading the newspaper can constitute a bedtime ritual. If you're back at the station after a stressful call, a hot shower or deep breathing and meditating for a few minutes can help you wind down. Even if you can't sleep, try to calm yourself and relax your mind and body. Have something in your life that tells your brain, "This is the time I wind down for sleep."

- **Creating "white noise" can help you sleep in the daytime.** Invest in a device that produces all kinds of pleasant sounds found in nature. These popular machines, which emulate sounds such as a waterfall or a rushing mountain stream, are available for under $50. Also, noise from passing cars and barking dogs can be screened with a fan or low-volume music.

Alterations in noise levels—such as attempts by your family to become *overly quiet* by tiptoeing around—will disturb your sleep. Shutting a door too easily can wake up a sleeper almost as easily as if the door were slammed.

SELF-CARE TIPS TO USE EVERY DAY

Getting better sleep, making small changes in stressful areas, and conserving mental energy will all help to reduce your stress overload. But take the time to see if you are doing anything to exacerbate your stress from the self-care aspect.

For example, many EMS workers say they have lots of coffee at work as a way of comforting themselves. Or, on their off days, they enjoy relaxing with a beer. Cutting caffeine or alcohol totally isn't necessary, but learning how much and *when* to have these stimulants is important. Also, learning to get a psychological boost from exercise and good friendships might keep you from *craving the unhealthy stimulation* of too much caffeine or alcohol.

It can be tempting to grab another cup of coffee, although your nerves are already jangled, instead of talking out your problems or sitting quietly for five minutes. Or, it can be tempting to have a mixed drink when comforting conversation from a friend on the phone would soothe you just as well.

Consider the importance of these comforting daily rituals:

- **Find some transitional time.** Taking time to sit and relax before work, between calls, before you go home, or before you go to bed is important. Having time to "shift gears" keeps your nerves from becoming frazzled.

  Beg, borrow, or steal transitional time. Linger in the washroom, if you have to. This time you take for yourself refreshes the brain. *It is up to you to find it. No one is going to give it to you.*
- **Think out loud on your way home.** Sane, normal people do talk to themselves. In order to avoid overloading your family, go ahead and gripe, groan, and worry out loud while you're alone. Say anything you need to. Nobody is listening but you.

- **Slow your thoughts down.** Once or twice a day, deliberately focus on visual objects—trees, pictures on the wall, anything—in order to stop your brain from racing. Switching to a different mode will take conscious effort. Pretend that you're watching a movie in slow motion. Absorb your surroundings. Look at the sky. Examine your daughter's delicate hands. *Enjoy the process of not thinking.*

- **Listen to good music.** Hearing a great tape of your favorite songs can relieve stress. In fact, studies have shown that good music has been a catalyst for change in clinically depressed people. These subjects reported less depression after hearing their favorite songs over a period of time. They found songs that were popular during their carefree years as teenagers to be especially uplifting.

    Why not buy a tape of the top 10 songs you enjoyed during a certain year of your youth? Play it in your car when you've had a trying day.

- **Have something to look forward to.** Each day, try to think of one small, inexpensive thing to do for yourself. Check out a book on vacation spots from the library, try a new flavor of ice cream, or pick up a magazine on home decorating.

- **Make a list of your own "stressbusters."** Soak in a warm tub, play a harmless joke on someone, or do an intense workout at the gym. Think of as many relatively easy activities as you can. Write them in the back

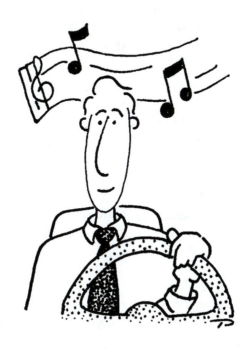

pages of your daily planner. When stress is weighing you down, find something on your list that appeals to you and do it.

Don't leave out activities that include being touched or hugged by other people. *There is no substitute for human contact.* Let your mate give you a back rub or play basketball with the neighborhood kids. If you're single and lonely, go to a civic dinner or dance.

Reminder

Burning out on the job happens quicker when you don't feel a sense of overall balance in your life. Relationships, hobbies, activities, and goals are all part of that balance. However, most adults who suffer job stress seldom seek help from a mental health professional until their marriages or intimate relationships are in trouble.

When any kind of life crisis is bearing down on you, remember to "slow down the train" and find out what control you do have.

Let's take a look at two examples of finding control in a crisis:

Job/financial anxieties

Amy, a paramedic on the West Coast, heard a rumor she would get laid off. She had financed a modestly priced home she was renovating. Her employer was being forced to cut back on personnel because of budget problems in their county. Taxpayers were demanding cutbacks, and their representatives responded by tightening the purse strings.

Before she started to panic, Amy decided to talk openly with her supervisor. "If the rumor was true, I needed to face matters right away," Amy reveals. "As it turned out, I was going to get the ax. So I asked my boss, 'Will you give me eight weeks to land a job elsewhere?' " She knew that it's usually easier to find a job if you already have one.

"I ended up moving to a slightly larger city, and I leased my house to my brother and his wife," Amy reports. "I protected my financial future by taking every measure of control I could. My brother even helped by wallpapering the house and doing some plumbing. Later, I sold the house and made a profit."

New dad crisis

Gary, a young EMT with a new baby, had just been promoted in his division. He was missing sleep to help care for the infant, plus he was stressed out because of learning new responsibilities at work. Gary's wife, who was usually upbeat, suffered major postpartum depression. "Let me tell you, I was petrified to leave her alone," says Gary. "She was getting suicidal. Her crying jags were unbelievable."

So what could Gary do when his wife's doctors weren't fixing the problem? "I called the women's health center and asked them to find someone who'd gone through the same thing," he explains. "They did. The woman they found put my wife in touch with a great doctor. In two weeks my wife was doing much better."

When you find your back to the wall—with your own personal job stress, health problems, or money pressures—it's tempting to think some person or event will miraculously intervene. But problems can worsen as you sit idly by. By assessing your options and taking some measure of control, *it's possible to turn most crises around.*

For instance, a responder we'll call Bill, who presently directs a large county EMS division, needed private counseling 10 years ago. "I was having crazy nightmares that I was ashamed to share with anyone," Bill confides. "These were not your average dreams about dead babies or car accidents. These dreams scared me so badly, I didn't want to fall asleep."

Bill was already heading for burnout when he worked a major disaster involving both children and elderly people. "This was the worst disaster I'd witnessed in many years," explains Bill. "Critical incident stress debriefing wasn't enough. I needed to see a psychology professional one-on-one, but I was worried what my family would think."

Bill finally called a psychologist. He told his wife and two teenage children: "I've decided to do something to help myself feel better. I found someone who can help me deal with my grief over this incident. I'm going to meet with a psychologist. Hopefully, he will help me look at things more clearly by helping me talk through these recurring nightmares."

As you think about taking a needed step, whether a problem is large or small, remember this: *Almost every time you decide to do something, there will be someone who won't like it.* But if it feels right to you—provided it won't rock your marriage or get you into trouble with authority figures (your boss, the IRS)—do it anyway. Procrastinating on something you really need to do isn't helping anyone. When your life is in harmony, it will help all those around you—including your patients.

It often takes intestinal fortitude to make a change. If a situation is bad, it can seem scary to change anything. Calling a marriage counselor, applying for a bill-consolidation loan, or confronting your child's ill-tempered teacher takes nerve. But if you're not an advocate for your marriage, your finances, or your child, who will be?

If there is some control to be found in a difficult situation, take it. Somebody may criticize you or even try to undermine your efforts, but plow ahead! Believe in what you do.

WHY BURNOUT HAPPENS

Stress that leads to burnout doesn't necessarily come from working long hours or responding to a large number of calls. Burnout comes from too much stress stacking up over a period of time *without relief.* Like straws piling up on the proverbial camel's back, the stress starts weighing you down. If you are emotionally overburdened, small pressures start to feel like bricks or two-by-fours.

There are many definitions of job burnout and how it overtakes one's sense of well-being. For our purpose, let's say that burnout is a state of psychological exhaustion brought on over a period of time. It materializes when one's positive efforts have failed to yield expected rewards.

Burnout can, of course, include many physical symptoms. Also, it can produce many symptoms that are identical to those of depression. For example, you may become easily agitated or feel isolated from others. Instead of feeling calm and in control, your anger levels may be so high that you lose your temper suddenly—almost violently. In fact, in a worst-case scenario, you may be acting out aggression on patients.

So how can you find balance? You can find it by learning how to reduce and manage your stress. You create balance by becoming proactive for healthy change. Once you can envision the coping measures you need, you can begin to implement important changes into every area of your life. You will begin to reverse burnout when you see that you *can truly fix* many of your problems. You don't have to settle for just coping from day to day. There are specific techniques and tools for altering those situations that irritate and anger you.

Having *the right number of goals in the right areas* is key also. For instance, striving to alter work stress, without plans to address family issues, is not a wise approach to curtailing burnout. Or, overfocusing on your children's problems—with no plans to take care of yourself—won't work either. Striving to find and implement balance takes real self-awareness. But once you understand how much control you do have, you can begin to take action for restoring your sense of well-being.

Positive self-direction

The following can help you understand how to gain better insight into what a balanced life means:

- **Get in touch with your professional needs.** For example, do you need a healthier work environment? Maybe you need to feel that you're making a difference in your company. You want to be trusted with challenging projects. In addition, you want to be around co-workers who are upbeat. Accept these needs as vital to your well-being. *If certain career goals or needs are exciting for you, they are not going to change.*

- **Document your personal needs.** If you need a closer relationship with your children, more time for camping or fishing, or a new love interest after being divorced for three years, etch these needs in stone. Stay in constant touch with them.

Whether it's more pay, more authority, or more creativity that you crave, be fully aware of these desires. Write these needs down. Although you may not want to write "I need a date" in your personal planner, do keep this need in mind as you plan your social life. Take all of your professional and personal goals seriously. Honoring all of your needs—whether or not they can be readily met—is emotionally self-supportive.

Your needs give you a sense of direction. Think of them as your North Star. *Navigate by them.* Feeling burned out can mean you're treating yourself as a robot. You may then begin to treat your patients and other people as objects. In burnout, you begin to depersonalize human beings—even yourself—to conserve mental energy.

A REALISTIC LOOK AT YOUR LIFE AND STRESS FACTORS

Have you ever had a car that you let run down? Perhaps you didn't change the oil often enough, or you ignored a rattle in the engine. You failed to rotate the tires. Pretty soon, it was hard to get the time or money to bring the vehicle back up to par.

Letting your problems stack up, without intervening in some way, is the same situation. Burnout intensifies. You might impulsively consider quitting EMS, divorcing your spouse, or taking some other drastic measure to regain control. But an impulsive decision can cause you more problems over the long haul. Address your problems in a more productive way. Think about a variety of options and small changes that can improve a tricky situation.

Obtaining balance requires looking at your life realistically. But, you need to back away from burnout slowly. Giant leaps seldom work. Change comes best when you make an adjustment, let some time go by, make another adjustment, wait for that to click, make another change, and wait for that to take hold.

> *Set the right number of goals this week, this month, and this year to gain more control and feel balanced.*

In looking at yourself, be realistic. Given *your* talents, *your* energy levels, and *your* desired lifestyle, ask yourself: "What's really possible for me to do?" How much can you accomplish this week, this month, this year?

Don't browbeat yourself because you're the low man or woman on the totem pole. Opportunities will come. Don't allow yourself to think negatively about yourself. Think about slowly making changes to get yourself to a better place in your job or in your personal life.

When you set goals, look at what's missing in your big picture, too. Do you need more education? Do you need a close friend? Do you need a surrogate family, if you've moved to a different state? By identifying what you need, you'll be more on the lookout for drawing those specific things into your life.

> *Your brain will access more of what you need when you tell it specifically what you want.*

Let's say you would like a promotion, but you doubt your leadership skills. Would you be able to gain respect? Could you communicate well enough to be in charge? If you tell yourself, "Yes, I want to be a leader in this department. I want a promotion," your brain—and the universe—will start helping you.

How does this work? You'll spot a book on "great leadership skills" at the bookstore. Your eyes will fall on a "leadership seminar" in the local newspaper. See how your subconscious will help access the opportunities you need. Buy the book and attend the seminar. Go for what you want!

Overcoming overload is largely a mental activity, but physical self-care is extremely important, too. You will get more in the mood to exercise, take a long hike, run, or sit in a whirlpool bath if you're programming your brain in ways that produce good feelings. As you start to feel better emotionally, your self-esteem should improve. When your self-esteem is high, you'll pay more attention to your body, your emotions, your environment, and your place in the grand scheme of things.

Developing the habit of focusing on what is going well is a critical part of having good self-esteem and cooling burnout. Keep reminding yourself of how far you've come, the hurdles you've crossed, and what is right about your life. *Focusing on the positive gives you the strength to handle the negative.*

PLOWING OUT OF A JOB RUT

Although you probably want to feel and act upbeat, are you in such a grind that you have resigned yourself to thinking: "I'm just another rat on the treadmill"? Almost every worker, whether an EMS care provider or a pastry chef, will sooner or later get stuck in a job rut. You're tired of where you are, but you don't know how to get unstuck.

Keep these points in mind:

- **Work often gets dull when you're not personally bringing anything special to it.** The trick is to find something new or different to contribute. For example, could you teach a class on handling communication with the family during a domestic violence call? Or, by searching the Internet, could you find healthy eating tips to share with coworkers?

- A career plan that includes educational opportunities, some volunteer work, and a self-designed ladder for personal growth is a balanced plan. But remember, the more rewards you expect from a single job—without adding something else in your life—the more anxiety you will feel when things aren't going well at work.

- Work itself usually feels more rewarding *if you're having pleasant experiences outside of work.* Ask yourself, "What is the quality of my life outside of my work?"

Getting out of a job rut means putting in some extra effort. But have you noticed how much mental energy you can spend coping with depression? Why not rechannel that energy?

Here's a checklist to help you evaluate how you got into a job rut. It's important to *reverse* these self-defeating behaviors:

- **Believe you're nobody special.** Just keep thinking there's nothing really unique about you. Make average goals and lead an average life. Never try to stand out.

- **Always please the crowd.** Never ask yourself, "What do I need from life and from work?" If the boss is happy, your spouse is happy, and your kids are happy, this means that you're okay.

- **Limit your education to a classroom.** Never pick up a book, read a piece of literature, or learn anything beyond what's required.

- **Cling to your comfort zone.** Never put any extra pressure on yourself. Do the absolute minimum you can to get by.

- **Refuse to conquer your fears.** Don't try to get over your fear of public speaking. Let opportunities to teach pass you by. Feel intimidated by computers? Stay away from computer classes. Let somebody else study software programs that might help your department.

If you don't have a plan for your life, somebody else will. If you do what the boss wants, what your spouse wants, and what the community needs—without stopping to make a plan for your needs—you've turned over the reins.

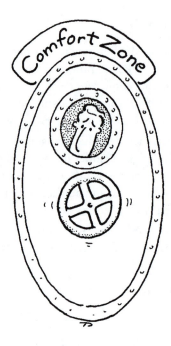

EMS is a great career foundation. In the following chapters, you will learn the building blocks that can take you higher. We will introduce you to EMTs who did curtail burnout by doing very creative things. In connection with their jobs, they pursued writing, teaching, and photography. We will also share stories from those who learned to manage stress and burnout as they rose through the ranks—eventually becoming influential leaders or administrators. We will also introduce you to those who have spent 30 years as an EMT—happy just where they are—without the stress of leadership roles.

Moving from burnout to balance takes self-nurturing of the body, mind, and spirit. If you're a supervisor in EMS, you owe it to your employees to teach them how to find that balance. You will discover strategies for doing that within this book. As an EMS professional—which is a very special calling in this world—you deserve to live your life to the fullest. We will show you how to handle stress, focus on where you want to go, and find those challenges that help you grow.

REVIEW ACTIVITIES

1. Name one small change you could implement today to help relieve stress.
2. Describe some of the creative ways people in this chapter solved problems.

3. Discuss the concept of self-nurturing. Why is it important to make this a priority?

4. What is the importance of having transitional time in your day?

5. Using the analogy of a train, with the boxcars representing your different areas of responsibilities, which areas of your life are overloaded? Could you think of one or two changes that might help to get you off overload?

6. Can you think of one or two self-defeating behaviors you need to address in order to improve your career track?

7. Imagine how an efficient person would tackle one of the chores, either at home or work, that you don't particularly manage very well. What advice might this person give you?

FOR SUPERVISORS

1. List at least two ways your stress increased when you assumed responsibility over others. Can you name two or three ways employees or volunteers might be instructed to do something differently to make your job easier?

2. A written assignment: Let's say that your immediate boss has asked you to mentor a new supervisor in your department. Write the new supervisor a one-page letter offering your best advice on how to manage work-related stress.

CLASS PROJECT

1. Have one class member pretend to be in a crisis situation. He or she is in full-scale burnout. Using the information in this chapter, have each class member offer the stressed-out individual one coping strategy.

CHAPTER TWO

FINDING THE SUPPORT YOU NEED

"*It was a cold, snowy February morning,*" *says Denise, a paramedic who also volunteers in mountain rescue. "I was upset because I had made an error the night before. Mistakenly, I had given incorrect information to an ER doctor about a female diabetic patient. While I was struggling with this pressure, I was also stressed out about my own family problems. My daughter had the flu and my mother was upset because I couldn't stay home with my sick child.*

"*Anyway, on this particular morning my partner and I got called out to a rather remote area. An elderly man was having chest pains. We risked our necks driving over icy roads that twisted and turned through the mountain pass. Our patient, who was alone when we got there, was having a heart attack. We rushed him to the hospital. The staff got him stabilized.*

"*When we got back to the station, this man's daughter called. I thought she was going to say, 'Thank you for getting Dad to the ER.' Instead, she snarled, 'Do you realize you knocked down Dad's mailbox with your ambulance?'*"

Situations such as this can leave you wondering, "Does anyone really care about what I do?" Dealing with tired doctors, coping with patients and their families, working out conflicts within your own family, and even battling bad weather conditions can take its toll. Lack of support from others can leave you feeling empty and angry. You don't want to be perceived as a hero, but it would be nice to receive an occasional pat on the back now and then.

Denise admits that she felt anger over what she calls "the mailbox incident," but she laughs about that episode now. "My husband threw out humorous cracks to make me feel better," she explains. "He said I should have told the woman caller, 'We didn't bring the ambulance. The roads were too slick. We hitched a ride on a dog sled'—you know, crazy stuff like that. Humor definitely eases some of the job stress."

If you have enough emotional support from others, you will learn to think more objectively about situations, too. For instance, when you are a new EMT, a good supervisor will probably inform you that citizens can complain to avoid paying an ambulance bill. Or, your boss can help you assess that an angry caller might be acting out feelings of personal guilt. For example, in the mailbox incident the caller could have been neglecting to visit Dad. Complaining to Denise gave this person a sense of being involved after the fact.

BUILDING STRONG DEFENSES

Stress management is a crucial part of one's well-being as an emergency care provider. But coping well is only half of the picture. You need to couple your stress management techniques with a complete "emotional support system." This system should be almost a physical structure of people, places, and things in your life that will help you feel better and stronger. This support can literally function as an emotional "cushion," which helps to soften the impact of stress.

It should include relationships with people who contribute to your sense of well-being. Also, having hobbies and pleasant activities outside of the work arena, an exercise program, and exciting goals add dimension to one's support. Even having favorite places to escape to, such as a hiking trail or a quiet library, can be part of an individual's support system. Anything that fills up your emotional "bank" with good feelings will contribute to your overall emotional security.

"There are two things I can't live without," says Robert, 31, an EMT whose long-term goal is to be a physician's assistant. "I need a close friend to chat with on a daily basis. I'm one of those men who does share feelings. The other thing I can't live without is a good exercise program. I'm single and living alone in a big city. It's been hard for me to develop a network of friends outside of EMS because I've been here only four months."

Robert continues, "This sounds funny, but I'm becoming one of those people who is addicted to the Internet. I'm spending too much time e-mailing friends, instead of connecting with 'live' people here. I've thought about joining a theater group to help build sets. I need some kind of new social connection."

Your goal in building support should be to look for a broad spectrum of people and activities. Think in terms of creating a harmonious feeling among the different aspects of your work life and personal life. In identifying your needs for feeling better mentally and physically, take time to evaluate any adjustments you might need in your life.

Ask yourself a few questions along these lines:

- **Do I have routines that don't work anymore?** Maybe your children are involved in too many activities. Could they cut out one afternoon sport? Or, perhaps some of your scheduled meetings at work are nonproductive. Could any of your meetings be fine-tuned for better results?

- **Do I need to get something negative out of my life?** This may be a negative person who's draining you or a negative habit you want to change. Remember that anything negative is subtracting energy you could put to better use.

- **Am I taking good care of myself?** Neglecting yourself will lower your self-esteem. Get more creative about how to squeeze exercise or healthy foods into your day.

- **Am I stressed because I need help at home?** Maybe you could "barter" for help or pay for small amounts of help. Offer to treat your nephew to a movie if he will rake leaves or paint. Or, pay a teenager $20 to vacuum and dust your house once a month. Even small amounts of help can add flexibility to your schedule.

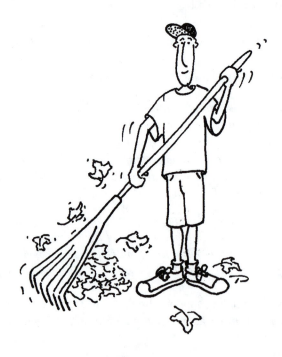

Reflect for a moment on these concepts:

- **Finding support takes less energy than feeling stuck.** The feeling of going around in circles or having your back to the wall, will use up a lot of your emotional energy. Actually reaching out for support is a better way to refocus your power.

  For example, if you need to plan your next career move, pick up the phone, and find someone to mentor you. Others sometimes clarify things that you cannot seem to figure out on your own.

  Even if nothing can change right away, you've gotten off of dead center. Reaching out for new information can relieve stress. It gives you a sense of finding control.

- **It can be tempting to *substitute* support in one area for another.** For example, if you need to talk with someone about your marriage problems, you won't find support in this area by working out at the gym five times a week. That's denial. If you feel the need to talk with a patient's family to obtain closure after an incident, you won't find relief by repeatedly discussing the incident with your coworkers. You will need to make an appointment with the family.

- **Don't neglect your self-support.** Staying overly busy by socializing or working too much *will not make up for self-neglect.* It doesn't matter how much money you're making, or how much praise you receive from others. If you are not eating well, exercising, sleeping well, or honoring your personal needs in some way, *your debt to yourself will get larger and larger.*

- **People who are positive and upbeat have stronger support systems.** If you are finding your life too full of negative people, with very few positive friends, consider that you may need an attitude adjustment. Are you in such a negative mode that you are pushing upbeat, positive people out of your life?

  When you reach out to a sister, mentor, coworker, or EMS chaplain for support, you will repeatedly find support if you incorporate a good attitude into your conversations. People who always have a negative approach to problems *will often lose the support they already have.* Being overly gloomy will make others want to back away from you.

Reminder

People who keep you sane and balanced are those *who validate your worth.* They help you to feel good about yourself. This takes having a number of people to count on. Relying too much on just one or two individuals will overload those relationships—causing them to deteriorate.

Professional's turn . . .

J. T. Cantrell, a veteran paramedic and firefighter with the Little Rock, Arkansas, Fire Department, points out: "Many young EMTs and firefighters believe they are coping by just doing more, pumping up their adrenaline and not letting the stress overwhelm them. But if they don't find more balance in their lives and have nurturing relationships, one day it will all fall apart."

Cantrell has experience in this area. As a professional with over 30 years of service, he learned the hard way. "I've got a wall full of awards and plaques for service," he explains. "But I sacrificed too much family time for my career."

He continues, "I could have made more time with my family. But in my twenties and thirties I didn't understand the importance of those relationships. One day, the emptiness closed in and let me tell you, it hurt like hell. At over 50 years of age, I'm trying to build closeness with my wife and children. Needless to say, it's tough."

In finding balance for yourself, nurturing relationships should be a vital source of your support. Your job, hobbies, or social life cannot take the place of relationships that help to ground you emotionally. When you have people to truly rely on, you can share your feelings more openly. With someone you trust, you can exchange humor, reflect on life's complexities, and bounce ideas off of that person.

Although it is important to work on your marriage, there are still concepts you need to understand about protecting your bond with your mate. Having good support *outside of your marriage or intimate relationships* will help those relationships to thrive. Different people in different roles will help "round out" your life, taking the pressure off your marriage. For instance, your father might make a great fishing partner, your neighbor might be a good companion for taking in a movie, and your EMS partner might be someone who'll listen to your financial worries.

"Trying to get too much out of one relationship isn't good," says Bob Mc-Daneld, former Kansas State EMS Director in Topeka. "I'm a firm believer that we should not do lots of sharing about work issues with our spouse or significant other. It will overload those relationships."

"People need other people very much," he continues, "but your mate can't be everything to you. I've been in a lunch group which included women friends, and I've also been in a men's group. Sharing with friends brings more balance to your marriage."

> *L.C., an EMT from the Southwest, learned this lesson the hard way. "I'm on my third marriage," he relates. "I used to come home and dump major stress on both my former wives. I used to cry openly in front of them when I'd had a bad call. I finally woke up and realized I needed good support outside of my marriage. Having supportive friends outside of a marriage is crucial. Bringing too many problems to the best marriage can destroy it."*

It's very possible to think your stressful job is fully responsible for relationship problems. Naturally, a stressful job often can be the source of strain between two people. However, never blame all of your marital conflicts on your hectic schedule or job pressures. The picture is somewhat broader than this. You do have a good measure of control over improving any relationship, even if your job stress doesn't change, if your partner is willing to help you.

Let's take a look at how a counselor helped a paramedic build his marriage back when he was on the verge of divorce.

"My wife and I were yelling at each other almost every day," says Chad, an EMT in a second marriage. "I kept thinking it was my work in EMS that was destroying this relationship, but when I got counseling, I found out that my work wasn't totally to blame. Our counselor said, 'Chad, you've got an opportunity here to create something you never had before—a great marriage. Get yourself a plan and act on it.' "

Chad continues, "The counselor told us that we could develop one new relationship skill per week. We couldn't perfect a skill in a week, but we could introduce a new skill each week. We learned to polish one skill gradually and hold each other accountable for progress. This kind of plan is actually fun to work on. It made a real difference in our marriage."

Chad and his wife wrote the following contract, with the help of their counselor, so they could tackle five new skills:

1. We will work on listening to each other, *until we are each satisfied* that we are both expert listeners within this marriage.
2. We will practice respecting each other's boundaries. We will work on this *until we are both satisfied* that we each respect each other's limits. A boundary will say, "This is what I can give or do."
3. We will negotiate conflict intelligently through enough conversation to clarify our points. We will not act out negative emotions. We will try to talk about them. We will negotiate conflict until we are both satisfied that we are good negotiators.
4. We will state our needs openly and honestly. These needs may not be ones our partner can meet, but we will each become thoroughly familiar with the other's personal needs.
5. We will find common interests that do not cause conflict for either party. We will build at least two common interests, so that we will have something enjoyable to talk about when we are together.

"In about a year's time, I believe we improved in about 20 areas," says Chad. "Sometimes we falter a little. Nobody's perfect. But one of us will say, 'Babe, remember our listening skills!' or 'Hold on! You're overstepping my boundary here!' It works, because we both want it to work."

Finding support for a particular problem, whether it is marital stress or work stress, might mean networking with people in your community. In order to locate someone who is knowledgeable in an area where you might need a boost, you can call a church, scan the newspaper, or call a large company to talk with the human resources manager. You might need to find a family counselor, a divorce recovery group, or a Toastmasters Club.

Supportive people are out there. When it comes to support groups, some groups are better than others. The personalities of those in the group will determine a great deal about your experience with them. Look for the right group, and don't give up until you locate individuals who will take a personal interest in you.

Kathy, a paramedic who wanted to teach EMS classes at a community college, went to a Toastmasters meeting to get over her fear of public speaking. "I was a nervous wreck when I gave my first speech," she laughs. "I actually got so upset that I quit my speech and sat down in tears. But the club members knew I needed support. Well, they let me die of embarrassment for just a few seconds. Then the club president said, 'Okay, Kathy, go ahead and cry, but you're going to get right back up there!' I did get back up, and I did fine. I've been teaching EMS for two years now."

HOW TO ASK FOR HELP AND SUPPORT FROM OTHERS

It is often difficult to know how to ask others for help. Finding the words you need to solicit a favor, a small piece of advice, or a pat on the back can be difficult. Will others think of you as weak or lacking knowledge? If you need to call a counselor or a mentor, you might worry that you'll be perceived as someone who is faltering personally or professionally. It can make you feel vulnerable to ask a close friend or your EMS partner for help. It can be scary to call a counselor or ask a group of people to back you up on a goal.

Remember these tips when soliciting help:

- **Know what people can realistically deliver.** Don't expect your friends outside of EMS to understand fully your pain over a bad call. Or, don't expect a new EMT to have the skills to comfort the family of a patient killed in a fire. Having realistic expectations about others is very liberating. It frees you to find support in other areas without wasting time looking in the wrong places.

- **Keep in mind that most adults have had their share of pain.** They will not be as judgmental as you might think. The counselor you might fear calling probably has his or her own set of family problems. The loan officer you need to speak with at the bank has probably been in a tough financial bind—maybe in college or during the birth of a baby.

- **Practice asking for small, doable assistance.** Make it easy for the other person to say, "Yes, I'll be glad to help you." For example, do you need someone to listen to a speech you have been rehearsing? Ask several people to listen once or twice. Don't ask one individual to critique you for two hours.

- **Give the other person ample time to carry out what you ask.** Try to give someone a day or two, or even a week, to respond to your need. Don't expect people to jump instantly to accommodate you. You need to gently remind people of your request. Busy people sometimes need a nudge to make you a priority.

- **Become adept at quickly anticipating what you need.** Don't wait until you're in hot water. If you're new in EMS, seek out a mentor right away. If you think you've made a serious mistake on a call, talk with your supervisor immediately.

- **Learn to get the good out of people.** All human relationships are flawed and complex, but you can learn to designate the roles of your supporting cast.

For example, you might ask your neighbor to attend a seminar with you, but you might reject the idea of asking him or her to plan a vacation with you. That's okay. Not everyone makes a great traveling companion. Or, your brother might be the perfect person to help you draw up house plans. But you wouldn't rely on him for financial advice. You know someone else who fits that role.

> *When it comes to asking for help, let's consider the concept of knowing what others can realistically deliver. Joan, a first responder, shares this story about knowing the limits of others. "I am divorced, so I coparent my child with my ex-husband who is also in EMS. We work together pretty well concerning our child. That's because we understand each other's stress. I don't worry myself about what my child's father can give or do. I know how much effort he's going to make. That keeps our relationship friendly and sane."*

A LIFE PLAN CAN HELP

Your stress levels will go down when you stop looking for support in all the wrong places. Instead of feeling disappointed all the time, develop a plan for your well-being that you know will work. For instance, if you're like most people you will have some "relationship stress" in your life, regardless of how great your associates are. Relationships need to be balanced with a secure "life plan" *that does not depend on personal relationships for its success.* We discuss outlining such a plan in detail in Chapter 10.

This kind of self-focus takes the pressure off of your personal relationships. For those times when your close relationships aren't working so well, it helps to put your energies into goals that are *independent* of your connection to others. When you have a good life plan in place, you can put your energies into helping yourself, until you feel more balance coming from your relationships.

> *"I put together a plan that included some spiritually uplifting things," says Danny, a veteran firefighter who was going through a divorce three years ago. "When I was going through this bad time in my life, I purchased a good motivational book. In the back of this book, I started making notes about small changes I needed to make in my diet, exercise, and approach to life. A year later, when I looked back at my notes, I was happy to see I'd taken a lot of those steps. What's encouraging about a self-improvement plan is that when you start feeling upbeat about your life, you'll start attracting more upbeat friends."*

WHAT IS REALISTIC TO ACCOMPLISH?

In putting together a wellness program to boost you mentally, physically, and spiritually, you can start by looking at what gives balance to most individuals. This would be friends, healthy eating habits, recreational activities, and so forth. But tailor-make your personal plan by asking "What do I need that is unique?" Maybe you love culture—going to plays, visiting museums, going to concerts. Or, do you thrive on rock climbing or water sports? Pay attention to what is going to satisfy you.

> Work on self-care routines, balancing your family's needs with your own, and goals that will steer you in the right direction.

Taking care of yourself will help you to take better care of others. You probably won't be in the mood to work on family issues if your own self-care plan has crumbled. It is hard to focus on helping a spouse with his or her goals when your own goals haven't been updated in four years. Focusing on caring for yourself will give you more incentive to give and do for others.

"Paramedics and firefighters can work hard to help and rescue others, but after a time, they may get fed up," says Robert Hemfelt, Ed.D., a psychologist formerly with the Texas Research Institute of Mental Sciences, who often speaks and writes about work-related stress. "This can happen because they're trying to fill a void in themselves that can't be filled from helping others. Something is missing from their own lives."

From these categories, figure out what might be missing in your emotional support:

- **Do you have enough comforting rituals?** Rituals help to ground you emotionally. Dinner with the family, chatting with a friend, or planning your next vacation are healthy rituals. But having a few rituals such as jogging or reading novels—which do not depend on the active participation of others—is important. When you travel or when you're forced to be alone, you will have stabilizing activities that keep you centered.

- **Designate places to escape to.** For many people this can be a local movie theater or restaurant. But for emergency responders, police personnel, and firefighters, this might not be the case. A universal complaint is this: "My immediate locale reminds me of all the calls I've been on. Everywhere I look I see houses, businesses, or street corners where I was involved in a scene."

  If this is your feeling, occasionally plan short trips to a city a few miles from where you work. A town just 20 minutes away offers new scenery to help you recharge your batteries.

- **Actively cultivate friendships outside of EMS.** Choose friends whose conversations are about something besides medical traumas and "fender benders." You may be in the honeymoon phase of EMS now, but there will come a time when you'll need to have friends who don't talk "shop."

  Remember that your spouse and children will tire of EMS conversations more quickly than you do. Many divorced police, fire, and EMS personnel report: "Among other problems, my spouse got tired of hearing nothing but talk about emergency calls."

- **Focus on things, not people, occasionally.** When relationships and "people problems" begin to wear you down emotionally, direct your focus to activities you enjoy. For example, if your brother-in-law's personal problems are draining you, focus on shifting gears to your environment. Would a browse through an antiques shop make you feel better? Would buying some bulbs to plant in your garden help?

- **Daydream about goals you've pushed aside.** Goals are uplifting when you're tired of your present routine. A goal becomes real when you figure out a way to make it doable. Could you break a goal down into small increments? Could you accomplish at least part of the goal?

  Goals give balance to your life because they provide motivation and incentive to keep going through the tough times. Planning new changes will help provide a new road to take you out of a depression, a job rut, or a family crisis. Neglecting important goals will make you feel you're driving on the wrong highway.

Steve, an EMS administrator, encourages his employees to believe they can find loving relationships. "There's somebody out there for everybody," Steve insists. "I hear a lot of complaints from single people in my department who have never married or they're 'single again.' When I was single, I couldn't seem to connect with anybody, until I did some work on myself. Frankly, I was unhappy because my childhood wasn't great. I felt sorry for myself a lot. But when I worked on myself, things got better. I worked on my diet, my goals, my attitude—everything I could think of. When I got my act together, I started attracting people into my life who have their own acts together."

He continues, "The girl I married was one of those people. She was not impressed with my looks, because I don't have any. And she definitely wasn't impressed with my paycheck. But she said I had an irresistible something because I had a good attitude."

In finding harmony with a mate, Bob McDaneld believes that it is important to make sure good experiences—hobbies, fun, recreation—are strongly woven into the relationship. "I've also found you can keep a relationship strong if you strive to agree on more things than you disagree on," he emphasizes. "This takes a conscious effort."

Making lots of small changes in your life not only will relieve stress and hopefully improve your relationships with others but also can help you look more attractive and think more clearly. Your self-care program of a good diet, exercise, vitamins, and sleep is your personal insurance plan for looking and feeling better. If you feel good physically, you're automatically going to feel better mentally. If you exercise often, your metabolism will be higher, your energy levels will be higher, and you'll have more strength to accomplish your goals.

Your life plan should include improvements for keeping you at your physical best. Taking care of yourself will help you take better care of all other aspects of your life. If you neglect yourself, you may feel too resentful to give more to your family.

You may be too uninspired to develop new goals. Maybe you have days when you just want to find a corner and retreat from the world.

Emergency responders should pay careful attention to the well-being of their nervous systems. The loud sirens, unpleasant sights and smells at a scene, sleep deprivation when calls are frequent, and exposure to traffic fumes and noises can leave you feeling your gears are stripped.

Pleasant stimuli from fragrances added to a bath, soothing music, a warm bowl of soup, a back rub, and even something as simple as remembering to soothe your tired feet with lotion once a day can help restore positive feelings to your body and mind. Try doing some restorative self-care things such as sipping a hot drink after you've had a shower. You may want to turn on some pleasant music and light a scented candle as you sit quietly in the dark.

Pushing for new, healthy changes takes a little effort. You have to plan and think ahead. You have to sacrifice time in one area to gain benefits in another. But most of the time it's much easier to change old habits and find new options when you realize *why these changes will benefit you.*

For example, consider the following tips for improving your eating and cooking habits when you're on the run. There's nothing here that you haven't heard before. But when you stop to think about why they'll improve your well-being, you'll probably want to give one or two of them some priority.

1. Carry a thermos or mug for drinking water and other fluids. Getting lots of fluids will improve your muscle tone, flush out your kidneys and liver, hydrate your skin for a healthier look, and help lubricate stiff joints. Toxins, which can make you sluggish or ill, can build up in the body when you don't have enough water in your system.

    Here's a test that can make a believer out of you: When you've felt sluggish for a day or two, look at the whites of your eyes. Do they look dull or red? Drink a quart or two of water over several hours. Then notice how much whiter your eyes look and how much more energy you have. Remember that water intake plumps muscle tissues, so carrying heavier patients will be easier if you've had plenty of liquids.

2. Make better choices at the "quick stop" convenience stores. Instead of buying a cup of coffee on the way back to the station, buy a bottle of orange juice or tomato juice. The juice won't give you a jolt like coffee can, but it will slowly raise your blood sugar for long-term energy over the next few hours.

3. Carry small cans of tuna and chicken on occasion. Buy small cans with pull tabs for easy opening. Add the meat to a salad at a fast-food restaurant. Although you probably wouldn't do this every day, it could work once a week. Once a week is better than nothing. If you'd normally eat a burger, 52 weeks of this fish or chicken lunch will save you about 200

calories per week or 10,000 calories each year. By skipping these calories for just one meal per week, you should lose three pounds of weight in a year. Besides, you would be avoiding cholesterol and fat, too.

4. Vary your diet to gain more nutrients. Toss a banana or orange in your purse or bag. Take a potato to work for baking in the station's microwave. Order sweet potatoes at a local cafeteria instead of always getting rice. Buy multigrain bread instead of wheat bread for packing sandwiches.

5. Vegetables should be a top priority. When you crave sweets, it's probably because you've not had an adequate intake of vegetables for a few days. Resist the pie and order broccoli or vegetable soup to go with your sandwich. Skip the candy bar and go for green beans or peas and carrots at your next meal.

6. Do allow yourself a few rewards. You don't have to avoid chocolate or candy entirely. Have desserts and sweets in moderation. Occasionally buy yourself a sinful dessert. But make up for it by purchasing lots of fruits and vegetables the next time you shop. Balancing your approach is what healthy eating is all about.

7. Use plastic storage bags that zip. Put a few grapes, a chunk of lowfat cheese, or small pieces of celery to munch on in these bags when you leave for work. Zip bags are more expensive than plastic wrap, but you can pack a greater variety of take-along foods in them. Baked chicken left over from a family dinner, nuts or raisins, a boiled egg, a small carton of yogurt, or half of a banana you've saved from lunch travels well in these bags.

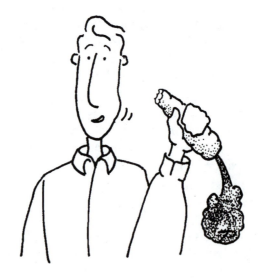

8. Take vitamins with one meal every day. Establish which meal is right for you, because taking vitamins must become a habit. Vitamins are your guarantee that you're getting the daily minimum requirements of certain nutrients, including minerals. This is no small thing. Few busy people can eat well enough to get all their nutrients from food. Besides, intense stress increases your need for certain water-soluble vitamins such as those in the B-complex family.

9. Cook in batches and freeze meals. We've all heard this advice a million times, but it works. Chili, beef stew, and spaghetti sauce are popular dishes to freeze. Make the chili healthier by adding lots of beans, celery, pieces of carrots, and green pepper, instead of too much beef. Beef stew can be made healthy by adding more tomatoes, potatoes, and peas than meat. Spaghetti sauce can be mostly tomatoes and herbs.

   Create a family feast quickly with the spaghetti. Cook some pasta, thaw and heat the sauce, bake a few potatoes and serve with salad and bread. When you're on the run, it is hard to cook for your family, but by cooking large batches and freezing certain foods, you can balance home cooking with convenience foods. Take leftovers to work and save on eating out.

10. If you're overweight, eat more slowly. It can be hard to slow down when you're on a hectic shift. But by eating slowly and fully tasting your food, you will crave less of it. The brain must have time to register the food intake. Try tasting each bite of food and notice how much less it takes to satisfy hunger.

REMEMBER THE FOOD GROUPS?

Understanding more about food will help you make healthy choices. Keep in mind that you need foods from these categories every day:

- **Milk Group—two to three servings.** For example, have servings of low-fat milk (one cup), low-fat yogurt (one cup), or natural cheese (one and one-half ounces).
- **Meat/Protein Group—two to three servings.** From this category have beef, poultry, fish, dry beans, eggs, and nuts. A serving is two to three ounces of cooked lean meat, poultry or fish; one-half cup of cooked beans; one to two eggs; or two to four tablespoons of peanut butter.
- **Vegetable Group—three to five servings.** A serving is one cup of raw leafy vegetables, one-half cup of other vegetables such as corn or okra, or three-fourths cup of vegetable juice.
- **Fruit Group—two to four servings.** Have a medium banana or apple,

Food Pyramid—Daily Servings Needed

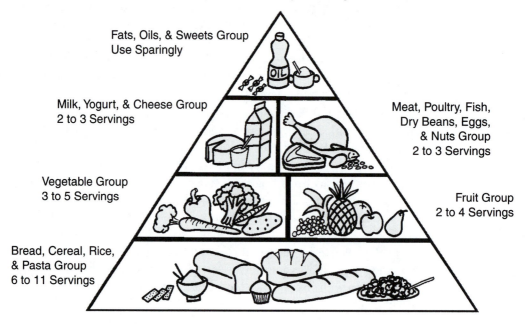

Fats, Oils, & Sweets Group
Use Sparingly

Milk, Yogurt, & Cheese Group
2 to 3 Servings

Meat, Poultry, Fish,
Dry Beans, Eggs,
& Nuts Group
2 to 3 Servings

Vegetable Group
3 to 5 Servings

Fruit Group
2 to 4 Servings

Bread, Cereal, Rice,
& Pasta Group
6 to 11 Servings

three-fourths cup of fruit juice, or one-half cup of sliced fruit for one serving.

- **Bread and Cereal Group—six to eleven servings.** Carbohydrates such as whole grain breads and cereals, crackers, rice, and pasta will give you long-term energy. However, the servings are rather small—one ounce of cereal, one slice of bread, or one-half cup of rice or pasta.

Fats and sweets can be a part of your daily eating plan, too. However, try to eat these sparingly. For example, three teaspoons of oil per day should be part of a healthy diet. However, most of us consume much more than this. Be very careful about eating too many fried or greasy foods. If you consume too much fat at one meal, try to cut back for 24 hours.

While eating on the run, it's tough to plan meals that include all of the healthy food groups in the right quantities. Attain the habit of visualizing how to assemble a fast, healthy meal. For instance, have a toasted cheese sandwich that is made from low-fat cheese and sliced tomato with a little mayonnaise. If you're counting calories, make it an "open face" sandwich—in other words, leave off one piece of bread.

Other quick meals are these: Have a peanut butter sandwich with half of a banana. Eat a cup of low-fat yogurt on the side. Or, have a boiled egg, half of a bagel, and one-half cup of applesauce for breakfast. Top this off with a handful of raisins.

For dinner, have a piece of roasted chicken and a medium potato you've baked in the microwave. Top the potato with low-fat sour cream. Drink a small glass of tomato juice to finish off the meal.

When it comes to taking care of yourself, there are four basic areas that you should never neglect, if at all possible: sleep, exercise, vitamins, and healthy food. No matter how stressful your life gets, try to bring these four areas into balance. Without them, you will become ill more often as the result of a *weakened immune system.* When your immune system becomes suppressed, you will become susceptible to viruses.

Exercise also boosts the immune system, decreases mild depression, increases alertness, and promotes healthy sleep. An intense workout utilizing weight training is wonderful for cleansing the body of toxins, too. If you don't have time for a workout, look for other ways to burn calories and keep active.

For example, if you're going to the mall, take good walking shoes. Stride briskly for 15 minutes before you shop. Or, jog around the school track while your child practices ball. If possible, park your car an extra block from your station, adding a few extra minutes of walking to your day.

Sneak in physical activity wherever you can. For example, make it a habit to do leg lifts or stretching for five minutes before your morning shower or while watching the news.

> *Joy, a first responder, told us she had lost eight pounds by exercising several times a day. "I did knee bends, side kicks, and push-ups against the wall for ten or fifteen minutes whenever I could get a break. I lost eight pounds in two months. Since the workouts were short and intense, they seemed to work better. Some of my friends said I looked like I'd lost twenty pounds, instead of eight."*

These tips can help you develop more incentive to exercise:

- **Combine exercise with something more pleasant.** For example, walk on a treadmill while you watch a video of your child's school play. Or, do sit-ups on the floor while your toddler plays nearby.
- **Realize that intense exercise will give you energy to burn.** When you get tired and stressed, your exercise program may be the first thing you give up. However, if you work out by implementing both weight training and cardiovascular exercise for at least forty-five minutes, your energy levels should rise and stay up for the rest of the day.

Weight training may not appeal to you, but give it a try to see what benefits it offers you. If isn't your cup of tea, stick to aerobics or another form of exercise that gives you both a psychological and a physical boost.

THE THREE PHASES OF STRESS

In defining stress, there are dozens—maybe hundreds—of definitions. However, a very simple definition is *anything that produces the feeling of a loss of personal control.* Of course, this definition relates to one's emotional reaction to stress. However, this stress can be either emotionally or physically induced. For example, a sudden change in your schedule can produce stress. Or a call from a telemarketer can make you feel angry and out of control.

Having to walk five blocks when you're late for a meeting, giving a speech, packing for a vacation, or attending a social event can all produce stressful reactions. Extremely cold weather can be a stressor also—especially if you must run calls in icy conditions.

When stress enters the picture, you will experience it in varying degrees. Depending on the situation, there are three phases of stress that cause psychological and physical changes in individuals:

- **The alarm phase.** During this stage of stress, your body and mind will mobilize to cope with crossing a busy street or getting a patient across town to a hospital. Your body reacts in ways to get you through the situation. Physiological changes can include elevated adrenaline and glucose levels in the bloodstream. Your heart rate can soar.

- **The resistance phase.** During this phase, the body's responses are in high gear. You are in the resistance phase when the stress is ongoing. For example, if you found yourself in a war zone for two months, there would be no way to escape the threat to your safety. Or, if your child is seriously ill, you are locked into coping over a period of time.

    When the stress factor or factors are ongoing, your body will become more sensitive to other stimuli. For example, when your body has mobilized to fight off the flu, you may find you'll become more easily annoyed by minor frustrations.

- **The exhaustion phase.** This phase occurs if stress factors persist. Over time, the body's resources may be overwhelmed. Depleted of energy, the body becomes vulnerable to fatigue, physical problems, and illness. The same reactions that help the body meet short-term stress can become unhealthy. Tense muscles can lead to chronic neck pain. Increased blood pressure can become chronic hypertension. A continual case of indigestion can eventually lead to digestive disorders.

Although having a stress-free life is an impossible goal, you can learn coping mechanisms and healthy habits. As you practice stress management, become aware of any self-help measures you might add to your list of coping mechanisms. Remember that "good" stress—known as "eustress"—calls for coping techniques, too.

Eustress is experienced when you participate in a sporting event or other pleasurable experience. Planning a wedding, having a child, or buying a new house are examples of events that produce eustress. Although the payoffs are desirable, you will still experience pressures and problems in completing these activities.

Emergency response can include a lot of eustress, too. Although it's exciting to assist with saving a life or participating in a rescue mission, you will still experience the toll these events place on your mind and body. An enormous amount of short-term energy is required by the body to cope. Be aware at all times of how you will take care of yourself in stressful situations.

> *"I worked three intense calls in a two-day period,"* says Murray, *a veteran paramedic. "Then I nearly fainted as I walked my daughter down the aisle at her wedding. I had forgotten to eat much for a couple of days. My blood sugar was probably low. I didn't pass out, but what if I had? It would have ruined the wedding. We can get caught up in our excitement and try to grab a candy bar to keep us going."*

Stress resulting from continuing uncontrollable situations has enormous *cumulative effects* on one's health. For example, those who live under conditions of extreme poverty are severely impacted by the cumulative effects of stress. When you examine your own life, try to develop a plan for managing your stress under such conditions. For instance, if you have a chronically ill child, you will need to develop coping measures for yourself. The cumulative effects of stress will catch up with you unless you have an excellent self-care plan in place.

HOW TO HAVE A MORE SUPPORTIVE HOME LIFE

A good job, a healthy body, supportive friends, and interesting goals to accomplish make up a balanced lifestyle. But few things in life are more comforting than having a supportive family. However, work stress can seriously impact those you love if you don't have enough coping tools. Some days, finding time to talk can be almost impossible. You may come home exhausted to find your children asleep. Then later, as you are going out the door to work, your spouse is coming in. How can you make it all work? How can you connect with your family for support?

These strategies are important for having a harmonious home life:

- **Honor everyone's needs.** Verbally support each family member's hopes, plans, and dreams. This doesn't mean you can meet all needs. But families that are the happiest consider a small child's needs just as important as Mom's or Dad's. Hold a family conference once a month just to say to your loved ones, "Let's all voice our needs." Ask everyone to share fantasy wishes, such as a dream vacation or cruise, and offbeat needs, such as more time to watch the comedy channel on TV.

  If issues aren't sensitive or private ones, discuss everyone's needs openly. For example, tell your teenage son, "I know that you'd love to have your own car. We can't afford one, but I do know this is important to you." Or tell your husband or wife, "I know that returning to school would mean a lot to you. I hope we can figure out a way to make that happen."

- **Find creative ways to build common recreational interests.** The old adage about families who play together is still true. If your family can't watch the same movie together, tape it and have everybody watch it during the week. Then discuss it over dinner Saturday night. Or, have everyone in the family learn a new card game or board game. Challenge each other to one-on-one games as time permits.

- **Remember that hugging and touching speak volumes.** A loving pat on your son's shoulder will stay with him throughout life. He will remember the hugs long after your words had faded. The hugs will be more long-lasting than the silly argument you had with him over cleaning his room. Your daughter or wife will forgive the fact you're late or impatient far more quickly if you remember to embrace her and say, "I love you."

- **Tell your family how much they mean to you.** People need to hear that they are important to you. Telling your spouse or child "You mean everything to me" are the most powerful words you will ever speak. Your family is not part of your life. Your family is your life. If your friends are your surrogate family, tell them how valuable they are to your well-being.

CHANGING BEHAVIOR IS TAKING CONTROL

When you are under lots of pressure, figure out ways to alter your behavior productively. Changing your own behavior is often the key to turning stress around. Do this by forcing yourself to make wiser choices. This approach represents self-support of the highest order.

Of course, there is no substitute for old-fashioned discipline and willpower. It's tough to come out of a "comfort zone" or a familiar routine. For example, on some days you might pull up to a fast-food window and order a diet soda before driving home. A better choice would be to order juice and perhaps take a quick stroll around the block before you head home.

If you want to climb a certain ladder of success, such as getting promoted or creating a fit body, make choices that feel mildly uncomfortable. Then keep pushing. If you take too long to get started, your chief opponent in this life—the clock—will beat you. A sagging belly will eventually lead to back pain. Or, neglecting your calcium intake, especially for women, will lead to thinning bones. You don't want to become ill in your fifties and sixties. A common lament in this age group is "I wish I'd taken better care of myself."

In your seventies and eighties, you don't want to face ill health when healthy people in this age bracket are now running marathons. You want to be running with them. Your checking into an assisted living facility because you've had a stroke or heart attack from eating too many fatty foods will be a sad alternative.

Try these self-induced wake-up calls to motivate yourself:

- **Sound the alarm bell loudly on something you don't want to face.** Write yourself a letter describing why you need to take charge. There's almost nothing in life you can't improve if you have a workable plan in place. Besides, whatever is negative will impact you sooner or later if you fail to take control.

  For example, your extremely high cholesterol count will catch up with you. Maybe you won't have a stroke or a heart attack, but your circulation could become poor. That certainly is no fun. Or, your lack of iron intake, if you are female, might not hurt your health, but you probably won't have the energy to learn a new sport or take an extra class. You will pay some kind of price for not taking control.

- **Try to raise your level of discipline.** Do this by tackling minor goals, until your willpower is greater. Get in the habit of reaching lots of small goals. These small goals should be part of larger ones that have bigger payoffs.

  For instance, let's say you would like to be an EMS consultant in a large urban area at some point. You're in your mid-twenties now. Outline steps to start supporting your dream. Borrow computer software that includes a career planning guide. Start laying groundwork to begin your own EMS business seven or eight years from now.

  You might start by taking one business management course or an educational course via the Internet. Remember that advanced degree programs are now available over the Internet, so educational opportunities have never been more available. One day you'll be behind the desk you've dreamed of. In fact, your present employer might be calling you for advice!

- **Break all of your goals down until the steps become believable.** You can't work toward a goal that you don't think is obtainable. If a goal doesn't feel achievable, or you can't picture the steps to take, try looking at what is stopping you. Having large roadblocks is proof that you've got more planning to do.
- **Resolve to remove roadblocks.** Ask: "What is really standing in my way?" Is there a way to remove this obstacle? Could you talk with others who have successfully taken a path you want to take? Network, read, research, and ask questions of everyone until you remove what is standing in your way.

It is easier to pull yourself out of a career slump or personal depression if you feel inspired by exciting goals. "Rustout" is a common term used in public health and safety jobs. As a new recruit, you might have envisioned EMS, police work, or firefighting as participating in lots of "glory calls." You were pumped up about making a difference in people's lives. But the reality is that you now have more paperwork than exciting scenes to manage.

Goals can help you restructure your expectations about work. They can be as much a part of your wellness plan as taking vitamins. Your new goals probably can't be as exciting as rescuing two fishermen trapped in a swift stream while the world watches via news cameras. No goals can pump you up as much as helping residents escape fire in an eight-story high-rise. But goals can excite you, if you choose those that can improve the quality of your life.

For example, perhaps you're in a "replay" mode concerning a bad scene or a relationship that didn't work. You play the same old video over and over in your mind. You feel stuck in neutral. New goals can help you refocus your energy. One or two long-term goals, along with four or five short-term goals, can do wonders in pushing you forward. Stop pushing the rewind button and press "play." Challenge yourself to see what happens.

REVIEW ACTIVITIES

1. Name one area of your support system that is weak. How could you work toward change to improve the quality of your well-being in this area?
2. Which three people in your life give you the most support? What type of support, either verbal or emotional, do you give back to these people?
3. What life choices have you made that you're certain have improved the quality of your life? Which choices have been negative for your career?

How could you change your negatives into positives if you really wanted to?

4. Name one choice you could make today that would have a positive influence on your mental or physical well-being over the next year.

5. If you could select one relationship skill to work on, what would it be? How would enhancing this area of your communication impact your present relationships?

6. Describe two ways you could work an extra 30 minutes of exercise into your week. How could you do this in a way that would be pleasurable for you?

7. Name two foods that you need to fit into your weekly diet. How could you painlessly implement these foods into your eating habits?

FOR SUPERVISORS

1. Let's say that one of your coworkers feels confused about setting goals. He or she wants to pursue more education; however, this person feels restricted because good child care is difficult to find in your area. How would you advise this person to work around this roadblock?

2. What activities could you plan for your EMS department to help employees' spouses and significant others feel more productively involved with your department?

CLASS PROJECT

1. Have everyone share the details of an incident at work or at home (without getting too personal or revealing names) whereby he or she felt emotional support was lacking. For example, have someone share how his or her competence was questioned in front of others. Then discuss how the person who did the questioning might have offered good emotional support along with the criticism.

CHAPTER THREE

LOWERING STRESS
AT THE STATION

"*I was under a lot of pressure a couple of years ago,*" *explains Gavin, an EMS supervisor in a large northern city. "I was spending all of my time managing the disputes and politics of three hundred men and women. They had more interpersonal battles going on than you'd find on a daytime soap opera.*"

Gavin continues, "I knew I had to lay some new groundwork. I had to start building a team out of these disgruntled individuals. An EMS administrator in my state advised me to tell them, 'Stop emphasizing your differences.' I knew he was right. Emphasizing differences increases tension among people, and dwelling on everybody's differences too long will cause a department to tremble to its foundation."

Gavin encouraged teamwork in several directions. He created a team for studying computer software, a team for organizing a fund-raising golf tournament, and a team to implement a new ride-along program for doctors and nurses in local emergency departments. "The tension started to subside," he reports. "I guess it's hard for employees to feel like battling when they're exercising more of their talents and having a little fun in the process."

If you are a supervisor, you may be lying awake nights trying to devise solutions to curtail the bickering and unhealthy competition in your department. A few simple steps won't fix everything. But implementing new teamwork concepts, honoring the rights of individuals, and working to have better communication with your employees should help. Last but not least, improving the physical appearance of your department and its stations can put workers in a better mood.

Upgrading exteriors, improving sleeping quarters, and remodeling offices and living areas are definitely worth considering. If remodeling funds are short or nonexistent, there are innovative ways to obtain funding and physical help from your community. Employee teamwork can make a beautiful transformation very feasible. How attractive and comfortable a work environment is will have significant impact on the emotional well-being of personnel.

But first, let's address the "psychological" atmosphere of a busy work environment. How can you create more harmony? Every group of coworkers has a different emotional chemistry, which is determined by what the group values and what the group considers important to its operation. In addition, the needs of individuals, especially if they are somewhat contradictory to management, will figure into the chemistry, too.

As a supervisor of others, you can rest assured that having to address staff complaints is one problem that is *not* going to go away. In fact, if there's no tension in your EMS or firefighting unit, you have a bigger problem. Either your people are collectively brain-dead, or they're suffering from enough *apathy* to wreck your department.

When employees make waves by challenging the status quo, it can often lead to needed changes. Perhaps your method of scheduling work *does* need upgrading— just like some employees are saying. Or, maybe whoever is taking care of equipment checks is not doing a good enough job.

It serves as a healthy system of "checks and balances" to have *some* interpersonal disputes going on. Naturally, there are exceptions to this rule. A few smaller, rural departments report that they have very few personnel problems. They have almost a family feeling among workers. There also will be weeks of relative calm in larger departments. But sooner or later, in most divisions, sensitive issues will surface.

For example, a stressed-out person might clash openly with a supervisor or disobey an order. Or, a medic's competence at a scene will be questioned by a coworker. And this "fighting and blaming" will not stay between two people. Other people— and lots of nit-picking side issues—will get dragged into the drama.

The emotional well-being of your staff should never be taken lightly. How people are managed on the job will affect their physical health, their personal lives, and ultimately their efficiency on the job. Also, your addressing complaints thoughtfully will benefit the financial bottom line of your department. Why? Because happier people show up for work more promptly and in better spirits. Plus, they will knock themselves out to perform for a supervisor who shows that he or she cares about them.

As a leader, you don't have to emulate a clinical psychologist, nor must you allow yourself to be used as a crying towel. But it does help when supervisors try to be *good listening posts*. When a frustrated individual has someone who carefully listens to him or her, it lightens some of the weight of any burden. He or she can *feel* the emotional support.

You don't necessarily have to agree or disagree on a point. You don't have to voice great wisdom or shell out too much advice. What helps is to listen, ask questions, and help the other person open up. Your employees need to see that *you grasp exactly where they're coming from.*

When you interact with a single employee or several in an emotionally charged situation, think about managing your own part in the scenario.

These suggestions might help:

- **Protect the egos of all involved.** Try to speak to employees in ways that are supportive, not demeaning. Even if you should have to fire someone, try to refrain from diminishing this person in any way. The minute you lose your cool, you have become part of the tension. Your job is not to fix all of the problems, nor all of the people. You can't.

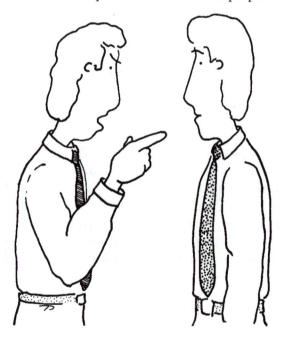

Your job is to handle tense situations with dignity, while keeping your own stress levels from going through the roof.

- **Let difficult people do most of the talking up front.** Don't necessarily jump in to intervene, unless you need to say, "Let's take this into a private office." Let those who are upset have the floor, as you nod and use receptive body language that says, "I am hearing you." By allowing people to wind down by talking a lot, they will be more open to what you have to say.

COUNSELOR'S CORNER

"Don't ignore a problem that's going through the rumor mill," advises Nancy Bohl, Ph.D., a psychotherapist who has worked with firefighters, police officers, and emergency personnel in San Bernardino, California. "I have worked with a lot of departments," she says, "and I counsel all chiefs and department heads to believe it when they hear that something's really wrong. The problem will not magically go away."

Dr. Bohl cautions that a tense problem should not be assigned to a coworker next in command to you if you are a supervisor. She emphasizes that the person who is second in command will often tend to downplay the problem or take care of it superficially. "This person will usually feel that it looks better for him or her if it's assessed that there's actually no problem at all," she points out.

"It's best for the men and women affected by the problem to meet, present options, decide on changes, and actively work together to implement new changes," she says. "But the chief or commanding officer must buy into these changes and actively support them, or they won't stick."

Dr. Bohl continues, "When I'm called in to help mediate for change in a department with problems, I very carefully talk with each man and woman separately. We work slowly and carefully to identify issues. *We don't pick out people to embarrass.* The one who is emotionally injured by the talk never gets over it. Whoever does the injuring never feels comfortable around the one he's attacked either."

Problems are best approached gently, in a nonconfrontational way. Head-on clashes, heated quarrels, and finger-pointing won't work. EMS professionals and volunteers, firefighters, rescue personnel, and police officers are strong-willed, proud individuals whose egos reflect high self-esteem. They are always going that extra mile for others, so they need to feel they have the respect of others—including their coworkers and supervisors.

Because of this sensitivity to pride and ego in the ranks, department heads must be careful to "contain" a smaller quarrel between two people. For example, when two people on a shift are clashing over a personal issue, gossip in the troops should be discouraged. The more "hoopla" that is kicked up over a two-person argument, the more each person's personal dignity is injured. Not only does the gossip hurt their pride, but it's also a fact that the gossip will muddy the waters. The real issues—which may be very important ones—can become obscured.

So how can leaders contain a smaller disagreement, so that things do not get out of hand? One way is for every leader in a department to take a strong stand on how the company grapevine is to be handled. For example, if all employees know that too much gossip—especially thoughtless conversation that could injure one person—is frowned upon by management, this sends out a strong message about the code of conduct expected of everyone.

If it's appropriate, counsel two of your employees who are having a clash this way: "I know you two don't see eye to eye about this. However, I'd like you to refrain from talking negatively about each other to the rest of the staff. They probably don't have the insight to fix your problem anyway. If you have to 'agree to disagree,' that's okay. Tell everybody you don't agree, but do not attack each other in casual conversation with your coworkers. Becoming grist for the gossip mill won't be fun for either of you."

TRICKY POLITICS CALL FOR DIPLOMACY

Asking workers to keep an argument contained to protect their dignity is one thing, but your failure to give attention where it is due can backfire. Issues that appear to go underground and die can resurface in a different way. Employees can "invent" new problems to gain attention from management when the old ones are ignored. Employees won't forget anything that is really upsetting them. Who could? If supervisors ignore the fact that some ambulances need servicing badly or they simply tune out rumors that a new EMT's skills aren't up to par, the men and women concerned about these issues may spotlight new problems. Pointing a finger at some new dilemma helps them feel they have some control.

Again, your job as supervisor is *not* to fix all problems, which is impossible anyway. It is your job to ask two quarreling individuals to *clarify* the issues so that you can clearly see both sides. Then try asking for solutions and input from both parties before you offer an opinion.

Write This in Stone

When a person feels understood, that person feels valued. This applies to a coworker, friend, child, or spouse. In addition, *a person's anxiety level will go down when he or she feels understood, even if nothing can change right away.*

It helps for the supervisor to support each person's right to "own" his or her feelings. This means that no one should tell another person, "Your feelings are wrong." Also, it helps to ask other people what they need, even if their problems are outside issues such as marital problems.

By asking a troubled individual "Do you need someone to talk to?" or "Would you like to share some of your stress with me in private?" you are going to make a real difference in the emotional health of your staff.

Many EMS units and fire departments across the country report they always use the written grievance format to cool tension between two dueling coworkers. Why formalize a quarrel this way? Some departments have this philosophy: If it is not worth putting into writing, it isn't much of a problem. The written approach forces the parties involved to think carefully about an issue, define it more accurately, and word their thoughts to take out some of the personal sting directed at a coworker.

These suggestions can help written complaints to be more effective:

- **Encourage the complainer to use "I" statements.** If someone says, "You always do this," or "You failed to do that," this sounds accusatory. However, if a written complaint states: "I need to ask you about a scene," or "I can't get something you did off my mind," the emotional focus is shifted to the one doing the questioning. All he or she is asking for are clear answers—not the "grilling" of the other party.
- **Stress that the grievance be fair, honest, and concise.** Require your people to write intelligently and accurately about a specific issue. Discourage their dragging in every gripe, groan, and irritation short of the kitchen sink.
- **Tell the complainer to focus on defining the problem, not embarrassing the person.** If a person's personality is the cause behind the problem, it will eventually become apparent. A difficult personality type can't hide in the ranks forever. Neither can someone who's not suited for a career in EMS.
- **Ask that a solution, or a couple of options, be submitted with the problem.** Have your personnel answer this question: "What would it take to fix this?" If a solution isn't clear, the problem's *cause* probably hasn't been well defined.

The longer the problem has been going on and the more emotional everybody feels, the *slower* you should move. The prescription: Meet, talk, implement a change or two, then meet again to check progress. Repeat these steps until most of the problem is gone.

The changes in a department's protocol are like the steps in a dance. When you've got a group of people working together and somebody throws in some kind of change, the group "dance" must change. Everybody has to adjust to the new steps. Demanding too many quick changes has everybody moving too fast—and awkwardly stepping on each other's toes.

INFORMATION EASES STRESS

Major powwows and written grievances should not be necessary in many cases. When people can gain more *knowledge* about a situation, this can cool tension, too. Giving your people access to information they need helps them to feel valued and part of a team. This information could be how raises will be determined for the coming year. Or, it could be information about new educational opportunities offered by a nearby hospital for pre-hospital emergency responders.

Reminder

When you keep secrets from your personnel, or they can't learn what they need to know about a particular call, tension will escalate.

Two or more people can have an "I need to know" session quite easily if a written grievance isn't called for. One person may choose to ask another: "I need to know why you stayed inside the wrecked car with the passenger for so long. I feel your help was needed outside the car. Two other patients could have used your help."

The EMT who stayed inside the car might respond: "I was caught up with what was going on inside the car. I couldn't physically see what was happening outside. I just didn't realize I should have gotten out sooner."

Supervisors should encourage their staff to seek the information it will take to satisfy them. Unresolved tension over certain protocols, or confusion about why a coworker was transferred to a different station, can be major areas of concern for some people. Personnel problems escalate when employees feel isolated from management or coworkers.

Frequent verbal support and positive feedback from management can help to ease stress. So can demonstrating to employees that their personal needs are important to management. For example, some departments furnish relationship tapes in the department's library. Videos on how to have a better marriage or how to become a better boss are available for all employees. One owner of a private ambulance company says, "If I have an employee who needs a Dale Carnegie course, I pay for it. Some of my employees have needed help in 'winning friends and influencing people.' Not everyone is born with good interpersonal skills."

In order to keep your people emotionally closer to each other, it helps to have a positive work environment and a *modus operandi* for enhancing pride, group loyalty, and good mental health. It helps to assure your staff that they each have a voice in what goes on, too.

Try adopting some of these policies for your department:

- **Stay close to company personnel.** Dr. Nancy Bohl says that a supervisor needs to chat informally with his or her staff, have coffee with them, and share stories about children and hobbies. A good supervisor will also share his or her past work history and open up about personal goals outside of work.

  Managers who won't let their hair down occasionally—and who won't bother to learn their employees' names—aren't going to have an overly loyal staff, nor one with high morale.

- **Encourage team building first and compromise for change second.** People who support team unity show more pride concerning their work and enjoy coming to work more. But having the right to negotiate for change gives them a much-needed sense of control, too.

The question your staff must ask about a compromise is "Can we have a slight change without hurting our team?" For example, perhaps a fire chief expects everybody up and fully dressed by 8 A.M. Somebody might suggest moving this up to 8:30. But he should first ask: "Would that extra half hour of snooze time hurt our team in getting the day off to a good start?"

Savvy suggestions for supervisors

- **Identify which problems deserve attention.** Don't try to solve every problem. Save your energy for the ones that really count.
- **Occasionally take a company "poll."** Don't *guess* at what is getting on people's nerves. Draw up a questionnaire that will document everybody's likes and dislikes about your work atmosphere.
- **Stress self-care and self-focus.** When a member of your department is exercising, sleeping better, eating right, and getting some fun out of life, this individual won't have as many clashes with coworkers. Installing workout rooms at the stations or paying for employees to join a fitness center are wise investments for a department.

Stress piled on top of stress can get to be a bottomless pit. But when people sit down to negotiate small things such as station duties, work methods they like or don't like, or something disturbing about a particular scene, it gives them some sense of control. Having a sense of control, however small, tends to lower stress.

Remember also that team solidarity is established when common goals are defined. Common goals get everybody moving in a similar direction. Supervisors should be team builders in every way they can. Always stress that an individual's needs are important, but tell employees and volunteers: "Let's focus on the common goals that will pull our team together."

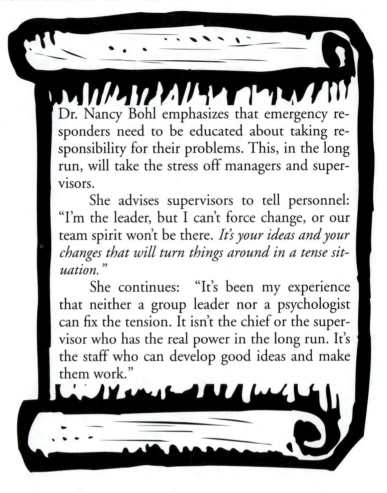

Dr. Nancy Bohl emphasizes that emergency responders need to be educated about taking responsibility for their problems. This, in the long run, will take the stress off managers and supervisors.

She advises supervisors to tell personnel: "I'm the leader, but I can't force change, or our team spirit won't be there. *It's your ideas and your changes that will turn things around in a tense situation.*"

She continues: "It's been my experience that neither a group leader nor a psychologist can fix the tension. It isn't the chief or the supervisor who has the real power in the long run. It's the staff who can develop good ideas and make them work."

When you empower others by showing faith in their capabilities to address the problems, you're taking a load of stress off yourself. Supervisors can become unnecessarily stressed out when they tell themselves: "I carry all the responsibility for change. I have to come up with solutions for all the problems." This false sense of responsibility will lead to burnout.

COOLING TENSION WITH THE BOSS

All the politics in any workplace setting can send employees and employers into a tailspin—not to mention sending everyone's blood pressure soaring. But one of the worst situations any of us can face is a direct clash with our boss. When an Indian and a chief are rubbing each other the wrong way, it's best to deal with it before things get out of hand.

Lowering the tension will take some thoughtful strategy on your part. Plus, you need to use behavior techniques that will help *both* of you feel better about the situation. The goal is to address the problem without making it any worse. It helps to get your logic in gear and cool your emotions.

"Work to find the source of the tension," advises Donald Howell, executive director, International Critical Incident Stress Foundation. "It's important to ask if tension is coming from you, your supervisor, or from both."

Howell, who is an EMS peer supporter in stress-related work issues, explains that sources of tension can be hidden, too. "Maybe a lieutenant has ordered you to get a burned baby out after a fire," he explains. "As an EMT, you may resent that this task was dumped on you. Several other responders were there on the scene. You might need to ask your boss: 'Why did you choose me to get the baby out?'"

Your supervisor, who would naturally be defensive when asked such a question, might need to be reminded why such a task upset you. For instance, you might need to say: "I have a baby of my own. I guess I just felt uneasy that you selected me."

The supervisor might respond: "To tell you the truth, I didn't think about that. I just selected you at random. Please don't think I was being callous. I didn't think about your baby."

When you can thoroughly examine your own part in the tension, you can get a better handle on what to do. If you can think of your boss as a whole person with his or her own set of stress factors and personal needs, you are way ahead of the game. When you take the mature approach of really wanting to see your supervisor's side, you can better judge *if you are playing fair.*

Once you identify the source of the tension, you can look closer at the problems related to it. For instance, you might be upset because a friend got promoted. You're not equals anymore. In a case like this, it helps to look at your own feelings first. Is your friend-turned-boss really flaunting the power that comes with the job? Or, are you envious because you feel you deserved the promotion?

A PLAN OF ACTION

"Once you've named the specific problems involved, you can decide on what moves to make," advises Darren Ellenburg, assistant professor of paramedic education at Northeast State Technical Community College in Blountville, Tennessee. "It's not good to ignore what's happening. You need to deal with it, because the problems between you and your boss can get blown out of proportion. Everything can start to snowball."

If your supervisor is fairly understanding and supportive, you might choose to sit down and talk openly about your feelings. Or, if you *are* wrestling with professional envy over a lost promotion, you might decide just to keep quiet. In the case of keeping quiet on this, wouldn't it be more productive to sit down and outline ways to make yourself more valuable to your division? By taking positive steps to help yourself get promoted next time around, you are focusing more energy on yourself.

People who work closely together pick up each other's feelings easily. If your supervisor has been absorbing some of your tension, your new focus on doing a better job should lower the intensity between you. If you decide to meet with your supervisor to discuss any disharmony between you, it helps to think things through and know what specific changes you need.

Reminder

When you ask for change, suggest some small improvements. Don't ask for the moon. Ask for what your boss can realistically deliver. Be sure to ask your supervisor what he or she needs from you.

Use these three diplomacy skills to help get the situation under control:

- **Ask to schedule a meeting with the boss.** Don't create *more stress* by coming in unannounced. By asking for one-on-one time, your supervisor will take your views more seriously.
- **Rehearse what you'll say.** There is nothing wrong with thoroughly preparing your message. Rehearsing will help you be more logical and less emotional. If you don't prepare, you are likely to say too much and escalate the stress.
- **Deal from strength.** How? Let your voice tone, body language, and responses give the impression you're a diplomatic person. *Speak your emotions. Don't act them out.*

  For example, stating "I feel extremely upset and angry about this" lets you keep your dignity without losing any of your impact.

If you are going to ask for some specific changes, it helps to know your supervisor's management style. This depends a lot on the individual personality. Is he longwinded? Is she a person who jumps right to the point? Plan your verbal approach accordingly.

It helps to let the other person know what options you'd like, but give your supervisor space to volunteer any cooperation. Keep the issues clear, but avoid saying, "You must do this," or "I am not going to be happy unless you do that."

"Keep the meeting positive," advises Michael Armacost, who has served as state coordinator for the Colorado Department of Health, EMS Division, in Denver. "It's important to listen. Don't waste time venting too much. You've got to hear where your supervisor is coming from."

The language you choose in dealing with your superior should be nonoffensive, positive in tone, and solution oriented. It never hurts to say, "I want to be supportive of you." Supervisors need to know they have loyal employees.

Reminder

Your best strategy for getting cooperation is to forget trying to change the other person and focus on managing yourself. *Avoid putting your supervisor on the defensive.* Don't push for change. Go slowly and act in a thoughtful, low-key way.

No one wants to help another person who devalues him or her. Your boss will feel less of a bond with you the minute you fail to value him or her as a person—or if you fail to respect this person's viewpoint or feelings. *There are no exceptions to this rule.*

So in a tense meeting, keep reiterating your support but clearly state: "This is what would help me. . . ." After all, you do want your meeting to be productive. Your supervisor can't read your mind. He or she cannot give you what you need unless you're very clear about what those needs are.

If the tension between you and your supervisor is high, lowering it will take time and careful strategies on your part.

Keep these points in mind:

- **Help your boss look good.** Be sensitive and be supportive of him or her, especially if it has been a bad day. Don't bad-mouth your supervisor to anyone. Speak behind your supervisor's back as if he or she were standing there. Voice some positive aspects about your boss whenever possible.

- **Suggest some mediation.** If the problems seem insurmountable, admit to your superior that you're fresh out of solutions. Ask if you can get the input of a third party, whom you both trust and respect.

- **Focus on doing your job well.** It's easy to get sidetracked by emotionalizing about who is rocking your boat. But keep your nose to the grindstone. It's hard *not* to gain respect from your superiors if you do your job well.

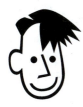 The bottom line is that your presence should have a calming effect on other people. You want your boss and everybody in your department to see you as mature, talented, and confident. So how can you accomplish this? Make sure others perceive you as a problem-solving individual who brings *stability* to the group.

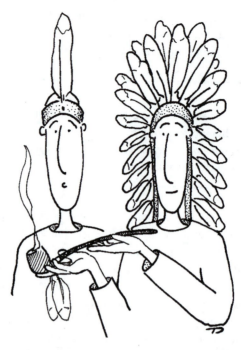

Clashing occasionally with a supervisor is unavoidable in most departments. Human beings are imperfect. Try to see that problems that arise merely suggest that some type of change might be in order. Before you get too upset about what's going on, ask yourself, "How can I speak and act in ways that lower the tension here? What small change might help everybody involved?"

VERBAL SKILLS YOU NEED

Whether you are trying to handle a patient who is stubbornly refusing to go to the hospital or an ER doctor who has lost his cool, you know how badly you need the right words at the right time. For many people, clever words usually come too late. If you do not assert yourself well in a tense situation, you'll feel angry with yourself later. By learning a few verbal skills, you can feel more in charge in many situations.

Try the follow techniques:

- **When you do speak up, act confidently.** Never act wishy-washy in an important situation. Lead people in the direction you want them to go. *Acting confidently puts you in charge of yourself.*
- **Listen carefully to your own voice as you speak.** Remember that people are influenced more by *how* you say something than by the content

of what you say. By tuning in to how you come across, you can make sure that you do present yourself in an intelligent, nonemotional way.

- **Use the "you think–I feel" method.** When you're being criticized, it can hurt worse if you fail to stand up for yourself. Offer a show of support for what the other person is thinking, but quickly state how you feel.

  For example, "Jackie, I know you disagree with my decision. But I feel my timing was right." Or try: "Doctor, I know you think I acted impulsively, but I feel my actions were right on target."

- **Cushion your own blows to another.** Let's say that one of your staff told the news media at a wreck scene: "The patient, who was driving the car, was clearly intoxicated." You feel like body slamming this employee, because you know your department could be sued. As it turned out, the patient had no alcohol in his system.

  Place a supportive remark under the person's ego before you criticize. You might say, "Brad, you normally work well with the news media. But your comment could get this department sued. Next time, get the facts straight and be more objective."

- **Help others to balance their emotions.** When you get in a tense situation, don't negate anyone's feelings. Fully acknowledge his or her emotions every step of the way. This gives you *more room* to be heard.

Your using phrases such as "I can see you're upset" and "This must be a tough decision" will show the listener that you are following him or her throughout the situation—not losing interest or looking for an easy way out.

Remember that you cannot fix the personality of a difficult doctor, patient, or coworker. What works is to establish control over your own environment. Verbally setting limits on difficult people takes practice.

These suggestions can help you keep offenders at bay:

- **State what you will and will not do.** For example, when someone is riding roughshod over your feelings, you can say, "I will help you finish this assignment, but I won't let you insult my capabilities."

  Another example: "I will testify in court, but I will not bend the truth." Or, to a lazy coworker, say: "Gary, I will make those phone calls for you. But I will not write those letters. That's asking too much of me."

- **Ask for specific input from the offender.** For example: "Brian, I sense that there's tension between us, and I know you do, too. Do you have any ideas about how we can fix it?"

When you ask for help toward a solution, you are saying to the troublemaker, "I won't handle this anxiety by myself anymore. The ball is in your court."

- **Clarify what you're *not* saying.** For example, "Tina, I'm not saying your performance is bad. I don't want to imply that at all. But I do feel you're leaving too much work for Tracey to do."

Difficult people see themselves as victims. They envision the world as a battlefield. Help them to see that there's no fight going on—just an opportunity to exchange ideas.

Reminder

Your challenge with difficult people is to interact with them without causing ill will or making the situation worse. Because this takes an enormous amount of practice, use a little humor in telling yourself, "Here comes that hardhead again. This time, I won't let him ruffle my feathers."

When you can deal productively, *without disturbing your own emotions in the process,* you've graduated to an elite crowd of great communicators. A lot of the game is self-protection, and it's your conversational style that will put the armor around you.

The following suggestions are communication tactics that are good to memorize. These tips can serve you well in lowering stress when patients, doctors, or coworkers are challenging you or complaining unfairly. Or, they can help you when someone calls the station to complain about an incident.

1. Never pretend to have all the answers. This is stressful for your listener. People instantly dislike those who pretend to have all the advantages in their corner of the playing field.

2. Be open to new ideas. Ask for input from your listener. After all, your coworker or boss could be right, and you could be wrong. A caller might have a legitimate point about the way you conducted yourself at a scene. If you have made a mistake, you need to know this as soon as possible, so that you can decide how to proceed.

3. Pause to let the other person speak. Listen twice as much as you talk. You will not gain one ounce of information by telling someone what you know. When you exercise your two ears, instead of your one mouth, you are putting more information into your own "research bank."

4. Ask yourself: "Am I proud of what I just said?" Scientists have told us there may come a time when speech from the past can be recovered! Let's

say that this happens in the next 10 years. How would you feel about the conversations you are having with those around you? It is definitely something to think about.

5. Besides talking and listening, there are two opportunities in communication. One is to build up the other person. The other is to tear down what he or she says. When you're exchanging ideas in a heated situation, consider which approach you are taking. Even if you have to voice a loud complaint to a sister agency in your city, tell the listener, "I'm not trying to cause ill will or tear anyone down. I'm trying to say there's a situation that we need to make a joint effort to resolve."

Let's examine how someone, supervisor or not, could unknowingly cause competition in a department.

To increase *tension among individuals:*

- **Foster too much competition.** Tell employees or coworkers that other teams in your department are better or more competent than they are. Or, try to "corner the market" with your own competency or skills.

  For example, if you are great at difficult intubations, you might feel flattered when a nurse educator asks you to teach in an upcoming ACLS course. But on second thought, you might think: "Why would I want to share my knowledge about this?"

  By missing your opportunity to share with others, you've missed an opportunity to promote goodwill between your department and the hospital. You have also lost a chance to make new friends and network professionally. Above all, patients may suffer some of the impact of your decision.

- **Always speak in terms of management and employees as "we" versus "they."** Build small fences—even thick walls—by talking in ways that separate management from employees.

  "I got so sick of our company's owner saying, 'There are plenty of paramedics out there I could hire, if you people don't like your jobs,' " says Jared, an EMT who eventually changed companies. "Our supervisor always used the same tactics. He'd say, 'The owner said to tell you guys this,' or 'The owner says management is changing a few policies about your benefits.' I felt disdain for the whole setup. Where I work now is a teamwork arrangement, instead of a hierarchy."

A supportive work environment isn't hard to create. It takes more personal energy and ideas than it does dollars to improve the emotional chemistry of a department. Even to the most eagle-eyed observer of the financial bottom line, the concept of treating personnel thoughtfully makes sense. Employees are a company's most valuable asset. Not only does it cost a lot to train them, but they are also a division's public relations experts. How they feel about their jobs will impact upon customers and every aspect of EMS business in the community. Enhancing their emotional and physical well-being makes sense from every standpoint.

Management can do many things to create a supportive work environment. For example, having employees' families to the station for a cookout is not only fun, but it might also help these individuals want to volunteer. Could they do fund-raising of some type? Also, family members of employees can help decorate living areas, shop for towels and supplies, or help landscape with flowers and shrubs.

Employees will respond positively to lots of small, thoughtful acts on management's part. A single grand gesture once a year—such as an expensive Christmas party—won't be as supportive and uplifting as lots of smaller gestures for personnel. For example, posting a bulletin board where everyone can share recipes, jokes, or ideas on how to get better organized is good. A suggestion box labeled "Ideas for Improvement" so that employees can offer their input might help. Management could pay $25 for useful ideas.

Managers can also develop a notebook with important memos, staff meeting minutes, and upcoming events of interest to personnel. A notebook with good articles and newspaper clippings on health tips is another way to tell employees, "Your well-being is important to this department."

Helping staff to volunteer in the community for speaking engagements or public relations work benefits everyone, too. Supporting the development of any talents and skills helps to "stretch" employees who want more interesting career tracks.

LIGHTEN THE MOOD, IF YOU CAN

Don, a supervisor of 10 years, helped to lower tension in his department by cooking for his employees occasionally. "The morale in our division wasn't terrific a few years ago," he confides. "Part of the problem was a previous captain who was aloof and a little hard-nosed. To show personnel I was a little less formal, I started grilling chicken and burgers for our employees just to show them I'm a 'people person.' At first, some of the men and women made a few weird comments, but I just kept on smiling and telling everyone to grab a plate. My occasional cook-outs and other changes have now produced a more close-knit work environment. I won't say people love coming to work, but I know they feel this station is better than it was before."

Helping to uplift coworkers emotionally takes conscious effort. It is easy to get caught up in what's wrong and what's depressing in any work setting. You can, of course, help to create a healthier work environment if you use humor where appropriate. As a new EMT, you can help some of the veterans feel more receptive toward you if you lighten the work atmosphere with jokes and a good attitude. The same is true whether you're a lieutenant or a battalion chief.

When things around your station or office get too somber, humor is a great way to lower stress. After a major incident in your community, or after an especially stressful period where too much has gone wrong, humor is often the only thing that will lighten everyone's mood. Humor helps to release hormones, such as endorphins, which boost the immune system, too.

Always caution your employees to use humor very appropriately, however. Ill-timed humor can cause more stress. Becky, a paramedic in the Midwest, had an embarrassing episode when she tried to use humor in the ER to help lighten the mood of her peers. Becky and her coworkers had had a killer shift. "Our station was like a funeral home that day," she says. "But I learned the hard way that when you're under stress, you've got to be careful with humor."

She continues, "In the ER, we were all concerned because this elderly patient was in a state of hypothermia. Her temperature was so low, it would not register. She was stiff and cold to the touch. We were saddened and appalled that she was in this condition, and we worked slowly to warm her and make sure she was okay. Everyone in the room was silent as we transferred her to the bed from the stretcher. We were outraged that anyone could let this happen to a family member.

"Well, my emotions got the best of me. I blurted out, 'Have her relatives been keeping Grandma on the back porch?!' By this time, this woman's family was in the hallway. I'm sure they heard me. My coworkers laughed, but I knew right then I'd be more careful about humor in the future. A paramedic can get so caught up in the tension of a killer shift that anything can come out of your mouth."

Clue in to good dialogue

It is important to interact well in a group, and it is imperative to watch what we say under stress. However, the skills for productive one-on-one dialogue are important to acquire. If you understand the basics of good dialogue, it's easier to have productive meetings, learn more about coworkers, deal with sister agencies, and exchange ideas with doctors and patients.

Talking with another individual is just as much of an art form as being a good platform speaker. Talking person-to-person in the right way is crucial for lowering stress in the workplace. The good news is that smooth dialogue is a skill you can easily practice every day.

Sometimes, we can treat talking as a one-way street. We deliver monologues, instead of having dialogues. We can be lecturing or rambling on when we need to pause and observe our listener. We might need to wait for clues on how to proceed. Making a point, and then *waiting for the other person to respond*, takes conscious effort. But when we don't listen, we're shutting the other person out.

Waiting for somebody to respond, however, can make you nervous. For example, you may have three important statements to express. *You worry that if you pause for feedback, you'll lose your impact.* However, pausing when you speak can actually make you more effective. A pause gives your message time to sink in. People will *remember* more of what you say, if they have time *to think* before you make your next point.

Consider the art of joke telling. Telling a joke too fast can blow the punch line. That's because a listener's brain needs to paint a picture of what you are saying while you're speaking. If you talk too fast, the picture will be fuzzy.

Good comedians use pauses to help the listener visualize. They tell part of the joke, then wait, then add a little more. That way, listeners have a "mental video" unfolding. They manage to "get" the joke because they saw the punch line coming.

Pauses give you time to bond with your listener, too. For example, if you needed to talk someone into getting into an ambulance for the ride to the hospital, you might nervously lecture, "Sir, please, think about this. Time is wasting. You've got to listen to us. Please don't be stubborn now. Think of your family."

This is probably the wisest route if your patient is short of breath. There isn't time for any conversation. But in some situations, you might need to wait carefully for a response. For example, an elderly woman refusing a transport might tell you, "I'm worried I can't pay for this. That's why I won't get on the stretcher."

By asking a question and waiting for a response, you could show an elderly woman that she has not surrendered control to you. Listening shows the person that his or her needs are being taken seriously. For example, you might tell the elderly patient, "What's important right now is your health, and I'm very concerned about that. Do you understand?"

After a moment, quickly add to this conversation: "Please realize that you need medical attention right away at the hospital. You need to be examined by a doctor. Will you allow me to transport you?"

If the response is still a negative one, try looking the patient directly in the eye as you speak. Tell him or her: "I understand your financial concerns, but the priority here is your health. Let's get you the attention you need."

Sometimes it's hard to get personally involved with others. You don't want to get pulled into their problems. But knowing how to have good dialogue can help you do your job better in any tense situation with a coworker or in certain situations at a scene. For example, good dialogue skills are crucial for lowering tension in domestic violence incidents.

As you listen to anyone with a problem—across your desk, at a scene, or on the phone—you'll get your best clues for how to proceed if you hear the real problem.

For example, Sharon, a dispatcher from Colorado shared this story: "I got a call one winter night from a man having an anxiety attack. He rattled on kind of incoherently about his wife and children. At first, I thought marital troubles had gotten the best of him. But, after I got a better dialogue going with him, I learned what the real 'last straw' was. The man's furnace had just run out of oil. It was freezing outside. The family had no money. I called social services and got him some help."

MORE TIPS FOR SURVIVING POLITICS

Learning to lower tension in yourself and others, plus learning to communicate well will help you professionally. But even in a life-enhancing profession such as EMS, issues of professional jealousy, misunderstandings, and fear over job loss can have employees acting out strange emotions. Sure, you want to play fair. But how can you handle other people who will rock your boat or undermine your efforts to enhance their own careers?

These tips can help you navigate when you're hit by a stressful political game that could threaten your career:

- **Try to never compromise your integrity.** There will be times when you must remain quiet, listen to the department grapevine for clues, and strategize on how to get ahead without shouting your intentions to the world. You must protect your own interests.

  But always think twice about compromising your morals under any circumstances. Losing your reputation is one problem that you can't fix in a lifetime.

- **Always speak about an individual as if that person were in your presence.** Your words will long outlive you, either good or bad, in a controversial discussion—however innocently or casually you speak those words. If you say negative things, there will be individuals who will shout your words to the rooftops. Why? Because those who fear taking a stand on an issue may think repeating what you have said isn't adding anything to what you have said yourself. This person may truly feel that repeating your words is just "backing you up."

- **When you're put in an awkward position, ask questions to get yourself off the hook.** Make the other person give information to you, not the other way around.

  When you feel backed into a corner, make it clear that you need more information to research the problem. If worse comes to worst, ask the pushy person, "How would you handle this? I'd like input from you on this." This buys you some time.

- **Don't pretend to have all the answers for someone else.** You don't want to be accountable for the life or death of another's career. You do want to help stabilize a rocky boat in the workplace, so that real solutions can be found. When issues become impossible, just say to cowork-

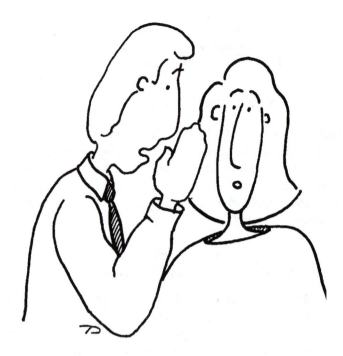

ers: "I can only be in charge of myself. I can't define the perfect answers for another party. I need intelligent input and solutions from you."

Here are some simple tips for ending some of your worries over station politics. You are the best expert on yourself, but think about these ideas and how they apply to lowering your stress.

- **Pay attention to your gut feelings about everything.** If you feel someone is going to sabotage someone else's efforts, trust your instincts. We all have an inner voice that guides us. When we don't listen to this voice, we can deeply regret it.

- **Sometimes, it pays to keep quiet and ride out a storm.** Look at the current political situation in your department as one where the tide will turn. Nothing stays the same forever. People move away, get promoted, and get transferred. If your station is typical, all of the actors in the drama before you probably won't be on the same stage 18 months from now. Focus on your own productive goals, not the drama.

- **Dodge direct punches when you can.** There is great wisdom in learning to "skate around" certain struggles, arguments, and negativity. If you want to rise in the ranks to a top management position, you don't want to be perceived as a battle-happy type. You want a smoother ride to the top. You won't make the climb if you use up your energy on petty problems that drain you.

- **Remember that you have only three choices in a workplace political scenario.** You can participate in and play the political game that's really going on—however you choose to do so. Or, you can challenge the game and accept the personal consequences—which can be risky, depending on the situation. Third, if things are terrible, you can resign or try to get transferred to a different work area.

Whatever you do, try to protect yourself without causing harm to others. Remember that you cannot fix people or force situations to change. You can only manage yourself in relation to other people and the situations around you.

Get support, if you need it

The tension in a department should be addressed as intelligently as possible, but what do you do if you need more ideas? Maybe you can't get a handle on which chain to pull. You want to do the right thing, but you can't define what that is.

Todd, a new supervisor at an urban EMS station on the West Coast, was worried that he was losing control. Several of his employees were arguing constantly. Two were threatening to quit if things didn't change. "A major heated argument broke out in my department twice in one week," says Todd. "I was certain I'd get fired myself, because it all made me look incapable. I worried that my boss would perceive me as weak and ineffective. What was crazy was the fact that the people squabbling were usually nice, reasonable, sane workers."

Todd continues, "First, I found support for myself. I called an EMS seminar speaker I'd met at a conference. I asked him, 'Would you mind giving me a little free advice?' This person helped me see that I had to foster support in my division by helping my staff to share their stress openly." The seminar speaker helped Todd outline a plan for change. Todd explains: "I asked my employees to meet formally to work on their problems. I gave them three pieces of criteria. I told them, 'I want you to identify the problems, instead of attacking each other. Next, I want you to write down the issues at hand, so that you will formulate your thoughts better. Third, I want each of you to give at least three solutions for what might help.'

"To make a long story short, the men and women finally clarified the problems. These EMTs and paramedics were staying in a bad mood for a couple of reasons. Four of them were forced to live in our precinct away from their families, because of our city's residency requirements. That's stressful enough. But all of them agreed that our old station was a depressing and gloomy place to work."

Todd's staff began a cleanup, fix-up campaign with a thousand dollars' worth of donated paint, cabinets, and wallpaper from local stores. "My speaker friend told me,

'Get their spouses and friends there one weekend to help.'" Todd reports that his employees' families did drive in from other areas to pitch in. "The men and women felt the support of their families and each other," he explains. "The bickering didn't stop altogether. There are occasional tiffs around here. But I'm glad I found enough support, or things would probably have gotten totally out of control."

LET'S DO SOME BEAUTIFYING

When it comes to lowering stress at the station, it never hurts to think about improving your work environment in the physical sense. Your surroundings can make a huge difference in how your employees and volunteers feel about their jobs. For example, in certain locales the personal safety of workers and the safety of their vehicles at the station are real issues. Does your station need more lighting in the parking lots? Should security fences be improved?

These concerns are very important to address in lowering stress among workers. But other physical problems, such as an unkempt building or a station kitchen that's outdated, can be depressing to workers, too. Poor landscaping or a tacky fence around your building can also have a negative impact.

Maybe you'd like to remodel your building and upgrade lots of things, but your problem is lack of funds. Your budget is so tight, it squeaks. Well, take heart, because you can have everything you need. Remodeled offices and nicer sleeping quarters can become a reality. You can have organized storage areas and a better all-around work environment. How? By focusing on finding the resources you need.

Turning a plan into reality

John Charlton, executive director of Washington County EMS in Johnson City, Tennessee, has learned to tap into other community resources besides hard cash to ensure his stations are better for everyone concerned. "I've remodeled and built from scratch several EMS stations," he says. "We've gotten creative and found all kinds of available help when money was tight." He cites this example for saving money: "Retired architects and general contractors have worked with us for a few hundred dollars each. Retired professionals are a wonderful source of help."

Charlton's department has acquired donations worth thousands of dollars. They've had building blocks, electrical supplies, carpeting, and paint given to their division. "Two people in our offices are very talented at soliciting needed items over the phone," he says, "and getting what you want is a lot easier than you might think. EMS and firefighting are considered very worthy causes by businesses needing tax write-offs."

A good example of such generosity is the Gray, Tennessee, EMS station that Washington County responders built a few years ago. Inspired by community need for a substation and belief that local residents would contribute, Charlton's staff got busy. Their total working capital? Just $82,000.

As their first step, they accepted a donated land parcel valued at $40,000. Next, they solicited almost $69,000 worth of gifts-in-kind—ranging from electrical supplies to roofing materials. Finally, these EMS professionals built the station themselves. EMTs and paramedics did everything from pouring the foundation and laying the blocks to finishing the interior.

Although you might not want to build a new station or to call upon your staff to provide this much labor, you can still have a nicer facility. Getting organized and planning well is the key.

If you do decide to think about remodeling plans, or your boss decides to delegate some type of station improvement to you, keep these points in mind:

- **Ask for input from personnel.** Employees and volunteers will be more enthusiastic about a project if they help to design it. When workers invest time and energy in the creation of their work spaces, they tend to enjoy them more and take more pride in their upkeep.

- **Approach two or three civic clubs.** If your personnel are already overworked, it can be hard to ask them to undertake telephone soliciting or volunteer time. Instead, ask your local Civitans or Optimist Club to help you obtain donated supplies and get them delivered.

- **Contact several office supply and home improvement stores in your region.** Write letters to district supervisors who are in charge of these stores. Be open about what you need and why. Follow each letter up with a phone call. If you are willing to pay a small cost to offset expenses, inform the supervisors. Tell potential benefactors that slightly scratched file cabinets, storage units, or bookcases are welcome. Your crew can do touch-up painting between calls.

- **Use the beauty of the past.** When you decide to remodel, keep intact anything that enhances your building's historical significance. For example, if you are working in a historic firehouse, try to keep your department's brass poles intact, whether you actively use them or not.

  Preserve anything of quality. Does your station have old, solid oak floors that would cost a fortune to install today? Why not refinish them instead of installing carpet or tile?

- **Place ads on community bulletin boards.** Business owners and homeowners alike may be prompted to donate office furniture, storage units, or kitchen equipment they no longer need.

  Advertise this way to solicit volunteer time from lighting experts, plumbers, electricians, painters, and those who pave parking lots. Emphasize to each that your department's funds need to be channeled into lifesaving equipment, employee salaries, and vehicles.

Even a little paint and some new furniture and filing cabinets can do wonders for your station's work space. New kitchen cabinets, beds and mattresses, or partitions in your sleeping areas might mean a lot to personnel.

EMS professionals need physical and emotional support from their communities. EMS administrators have a great opportunity to solicit this support. Hospitals can be encouraged to have an "EMS Appreciation Day." Local artists can be encouraged to lend or donate paintings to EMS and fire stations. Citizens can be encouraged to share past copies of health magazines or books on travel with employees.

Creating a better work environment, both emotionally and physically, will take lots of small, manageable steps. No one ever changed the chemistry of any workplace setting overnight. But you can have what your staff considers important—a new workout room, a well-stocked library, new kitchen appliances, or an on-premises picnic area for employees and their families.

"Don't worry that you can't make it happen," says John Charlton. "Get creative with your ideas, solicit what you need and stick to your plans. *Others will jump on your bandwagon if you believe in it.*"

REVIEW ACTIVITIES

1. If a coworker did something unprofessional in a critical triage situation, what would be the best way to confront him or her? For example, how could you address the situation without making things worse for either of you?

2. When someone has upset you, why is it helpful to thoroughly rehearse what you will say to him or her?

3. Consider this: You've just gotten the news that your friend has received a promotion. You'll be answering directly to her. You are extremely upset, because you secretly felt you would get the promotion. How can you handle your frustration? Would you still be able to feel close to this individual?

4. If you need to confront a subordinate about the rude way he behaved on the phone, what voice tone and body language should you use?

5. What verbal response would be appropriate if you learned through the grapevine that someone had questioned your competence at a scene?

6. If you were put in charge of upgrading a station's work environment, why would it be productive to take a poll among employees concerning priorities?

7. What five things do you believe are most important for any worker to feel good about in his or her physical work environment?

For Supervisors

1. If a new employee challenged one of your decisions in front of others, what kind of voice tone and mannerisms would make you look out of control? Describe the type of body language and verbal approach a respected leader might use.

2. Let's say that your department's work atmosphere is beginning to feel very negatively charged. Everyone is complaining too much. How could you create a plan to turn things around? What kind of goals would be productive in this situation? How could you foster teamwork instead of competition?

Class Project

1. Try role-playing a tense situation. Have one member of the class pretend the boss has just given him or her a stern reprimand. The boss has accused this individual of talking about a coworker in a negative way. Have two other students help this person calm down and respond appropriately to the situation. Then have all class members discuss how the person who was reprimanded might talk further with the boss.

    The goal in role playing: The class should help the stressed individual to *balance his or her emotions* while dealing with the pressures of a tense situation with a supervisor.

CHAPTER FOUR

KILLER JOB STRESS

If you have been in emergency response for any length of time, you probably have experienced some form of depression. For a period of time, you might have had trouble eating, sleeping, and thinking clearly. Maybe your doctor prescribed a tranquilizer or sleeping aid. You took a week's vacation, extended by some personal leave days. During this time away from work, you experienced a change of scenery, increased your rest, and began to feel better. Your blue feeling eventually lifted. You were back to your old self.

But what if you are locked into a depression that isn't going away? Let's say that you worked a car crash incident two months ago. Two children were killed who reminded you of your own. A few days later, you helped recover two bodies in a drowning incident. One of the victims was a former high school classmate. To top things off, this week you were called to a railroad crossing scene. An elderly woman was dismembered. Her face was remarkably similar to your own grandmother's. When you looked in the mirror this morning, you told yourself, "I'm coming apart at the seams."

You may be experiencing nightmares so terrifying that you are afraid to fall asleep. Your thoughts during the daytime are weird—even a little crazy. You feel spacey, disconnected from other people. Life looks hopeless, and your motivation is zero. Coping with routine job stress has been difficult enough. Now you have such overwhelming stress that you're wondering if your sanity is at stake.

How can you deal with it all? You have considered asking for Critical Incident Stress Debriefing (CISD). But would that do any good? You have thought about calling a private counselor. But what would your family say? Would your boss and coworkers have to know? Reaching out for help can seem as equally overwhelming as the stress itself.

Whether or not you immediately request CISD or private counseling, the following suggestions can help you find a small measure of control right away:

- **Find an active listener.** If you have not picked up the phone to obtain formal counseling, you should at least get some *immediate support.* Don't rely on casual conversation with a coworker or your best friend. Find an "authority figure" who is educated in how to listen actively and offer good feedback.

  This person could be a social worker in your area. Or, support could come from a psychologist who will agree to speak with you by phone. A peer supporter trained to assist you or an EMS chaplain who will meet with you after work can also help. A person trained to offer support in a crisis will help you feel you're not alone with your burden.

- **Avoid extreme thinking.** For example, if a child abuse call is getting you down, you could tell yourself, "The world is a mess. People are crazy. Our society is not worth anything." These thoughts are normal for anyone in your shoes. But try to get off this track. Extreme thinking will cause your brain to conjure up all kinds of negative associations.

- **Stop rehearsing negative thoughts.** Repeating depressing thoughts over and over will cause anyone to become somewhat depressed, even if they have no threatening problems. Picture a negative thought as a shovel you're using to dig yourself in deeper. Try to talk to yourself in slightly more positive ways.

  For example, you could say, "I feel awful, but this is not going to last forever. Others have recovered from depression. I can, too."

- **Consider the power of "thought stoppage."** One example of this is a technique that involves wearing a rubber band around your wrist. When a bad thought or bad scene enters your mind, you flick the rubber band hard and say, "No!"

  Although this won't work for generalized anxiety or complex problems that are bothering you, thought stoppage can work well on preventing a *single disturbing idea or scene* from pervading your thoughts. Try it for a minimum of two to three days to get good results.

- **Locate the name of at least two excellent counselors now.** When you are under severe stress, it pays to start finding therapists in your area who are trained to help police, fire, and EMS professionals. If possible, do some research to find out if these counselors are highly recommended. You can always figure out a way to do this discreetly. If you have to tell others, "I need this information for a friend," that's fine. Make a few calls or ask someone you trust, such as a chaplain or police captain outside of EMS, to help you target a good therapist.

If you wait until you're in a true crisis—feeling suicidal, having intense crying spells—you're not going to feel like checking references. Get at least two names, preferably more, because a counselor can be heavily booked for months.

Gabe, a paramedic who worked a bombing incident in a large city several years ago says, "I got into counseling with a young and inexperienced therapist. My counselor didn't know how to deal with critical incident stress. I was in too much pain to notice which counselor my public mental health agency chose for me. This counselor had lots of empathy, but no expertise on how to guide me. Finally, I told the agency's director, 'Please find me a counselor who's dealt with problems similar to mine.' After doing some fact checking, this director sent me to an excellent counselor."

Lee, a shift supervisor at a metropolitan rescue squad, worked a major airline crash a few years ago. He shares this story: "The crash bothered me for months. I had nightmares and full-blown panic attacks. Out of the blue, I'd start hyperventilating. Then I'd start trembling and sweating. I think the incident triggered every bad memory I had from my Vietnam days. I was terrified of being alone. I'd call my wife at work and beg her to come home early to be with me."

Lee explains: "For weeks, I was in a foggy state—you know, that kind of mental blur where you drive home but you can't remember how you got there. Well, one

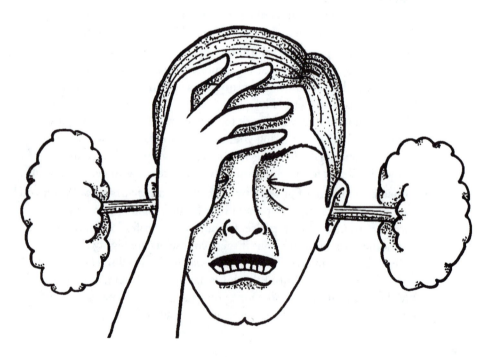

day, I drove 'home'—to a house we had lived in three years before! That woke me up. That day I called our local mental health agency and made an appointment."

WHEN PRIVATE COUNSELING PAYS

If your major symptoms haven't improved after three weeks, it is important to seek individual therapy. Going for counseling shows strength and intelligence. We don't live in the Stone Age anymore. Only a very uninformed individual would see therapy as a weakness. Asking for help should be perceived as part of your wellness program.

Keep in mind that most people who seek counseling are very sane, balanced individuals who need objective feedback in putting their problems into perspective. They don't need "fixing." They need a professional person to "share" their stress.

They need someone to help them decide what is important, what's not, and how to let the unimportant things go. They need someone to help them define a bottom line about how to view stressful problems.

> *"Whatever pulls you out of a depression must be powerful enough to do the job,"* advises Brent, a 37-year-old responder who worked a flood that killed over 100 people. *"If your car was stuck in the mud, you wouldn't use a flimsy rope to pull it out. You'd use a strong chain. Private counseling is like a chain that will get you out of the hole."*
>
> Brent goes on to say that he believes a chain of support must include several *"links"* of assistance besides a counselor. *"I needed my wife and my EMS partner to listen to me almost every day between counseling sessions. They were wonderful about my unloading on them. Another link in my chain was vigorous exercise. I ran or swam several times a week.*
>
> *"I also used writing as therapy. When I couldn't sleep, I'd get up and write down my feelings—the anger, the fear, the thoughts of helplessness—and then I'd tear up the paper. Writing is excellent therapy when you don't have anyone to call."*

Suicidal thoughts are very common in emergency workers who've been depressed for some time. If it has been at least six months since you've felt well, you are probably feeling very "spaced-out" at times. It is common to think you have gone a little over the edge. These problems largely can be due to physiological changes. For example, when you have lots of interrupted sleep, you won't enter the deeper phase of sleep where dreaming occurs.

Without entering this deeper state of the sleep cycle, your brain will not manufacture important hormones your body needs. This sleep deprivation can affect how you think and feel. Also, major depression can lead to poor eating habits or no appetite, which can disturb the body's blood sugar levels. Even mild hypoglycemia can intensify anxiety. Major stress will cause you to be so symptomatic that it will be hard to distinguish biological from psychological symptoms.

> *"After I got into therapy, I realized that I should have gotten there a lot sooner,"* says Jody, 40, a paramedic instructor from Canada. *"My therapist helped me feel I had control buttons. Before counseling, I felt like somebody trapped in one of those spaceships in a movie. You know, the part where one of the actors says, 'All systems are down. We're spinning out of control.' "*

When it comes to finding more personal control buttons to push, every individual must figure out his or her own. Talking openly with a good counselor will help you to uncover what those control measures will be. Therapy works differently for every individual, but personal counseling can offer these kinds of benefits:

- **Therapy can help you figure out if past issues are prolonging your pain.** Almost all adults have some emotional baggage left over from childhood. We all have issues from the past that need to be addressed. We must separate ourselves from these problems, so that this baggage doesn't weigh our lives down in the present.

  For example, you might be reacting strongly to a domestic violence call because your own childhood family struggled with such problems. Just recognizing and reflecting on this fact can help you deal differently with job stress.

  > *"I greatly overreacted to a lot of calls because my own father was abusive,"* says Ginger, a first responder. *"In therapy, I began to understand that seeing myself as a victim kept me in a child's role—a helpless role. I learned to forgive my father over a long period of time."*

  > She continues, *"What was happening with my calls was that every time I had to deal with an elderly person or a child, I'd think: 'Somebody here is neglecting somebody. This shouldn't have happened.' Then I'd get angry and spend hours reacting. Therapy helped me stop dragging my own past into my work."*

- **Counseling can help you compartmentalize your worries.** When you first go to counseling sessions, you will probably have all of your troubles—financial stress, parenting worries, work issues, marital tension— lumped into one big basket. Carrying that huge basket has overwhelmed your nervous system.

  In therapy, you will learn to put your problems into smaller baskets. You will learn to break problems down into smaller, bite-size pieces where they can be managed.

- **A counselor can help you see the larger picture.** Staying lost in your own thinking too much will eventually cause you to lose perspective on life's greater pleasures. Sad and depressed thinking is a narrow kind of focus. In this state, you can forget about how you fit into the grand scheme of things. Depression makes you feel locked into a very small room with no way out.

Your goal in counseling isn't to arrive at a place where sad events have no significance for you. Nor is your goal necessarily to become a shouting optimist. Your goal is to look at life from a larger perspective from which you don't feel so overwhelmed by one or two incidents. You want to find a more neutral "safe place" for yourself.

For example, by talking things out after a child abuse call, you might reflect on it this way: "I despise what this parent did, but I have to focus on *my* role. Did I carry out my role, however limited, in the best way I could? Did I focus on helping the child, instead of reacting too much? I don't want to become paralyzed by child abuse events. If I do that, I won't be able to help the next child."

A good counselor can help you deal with your depression from several perspectives, but you will recover much faster if you actively participate in your own recovery. This cannot be overemphasized. *You have to want to get well.* No therapist can do your work for you. You have choices on how you will hasten your recovery.

> *For example, Gayle, a psychologist from the Midwest, points out: "Some clients fail to understand one important principal about therapy: Talking about your problems enough each day will help you get well. Talking about them too much will increase your stress.*
>
> *"I've had clients who didn't know how wonderful it was to have a good listener— until they met me," she laughs. "Some would tell me all of their problems quickly. This was great. We'd really started to make progress. But then these clients would go out of my office and rehearse their problems over and over, maybe talking to their friends two or three hours a day on the phone about their troubles. This is normal the first two or three weeks. But later, this is not the way to go! Focusing on other positive areas of life, even during intense counseling, is necessary."*

If you are considering counseling, you may choose to share or not share this decision with others. It is totally up to you. Depending on how supportive your family and coworkers are, you might decide to be very open about it. Or, you might choose to confide in only one or two people.

For the most part, sharing with coworkers will probably be a positive move. They will realize they could easily be in your shoes. When it comes to telling your boss, however, remember that it can be a little more involved. It can be a tense moment when you tell your boss, "I'm not coping well. I need help."

That's why you should share your decision to obtain counseling with a spouse, friend, or counselor on the phone first. Then tell your boss. Get your feelings about going for help out in the open with a confidante or two, until you're comfortable sharing this information. This sharing will release some of the pressure before you meet with your supervisor.

When you decide to go for counseling, you will need to ask your boss if your department will pay for it. If you are in a large urban division, all of your expenses will probably be covered by the Employee Assistance Program. But even if you work in a rural area with a limited budget as a volunteer, counseling is always available through a county mental health agency.

Such agencies charge fees based on your ability to pay. Often this is less than $20 per visit. Because your stress is work related, however, your department should pick up the expenses. But never assume that it will. Ask your supervisor first.

When you do break the news to your boss, get right to the point. For example, you could say, "I have stress that's become unmanageable due to some of the calls I've worked. I feel I could benefit from private counseling." Act confident about your decision and make good eye contact as you speak. You don't need to go into details about your symptoms. That's your personal business.

Be clear about the options you have already tried. Tell your supervisor if you have tried peer counseling, Critical Incident Stress Debriefing, talking with a clergyman, or sharing with coworkers. You want your boss to understand that you've exhausted your usual resources. Let there be no doubt that private counseling is your next choice.

You might want to ask your supervisor if he or she could recommend a good therapist. Or, you can use the Yellow Pages to find local mental health agencies. Agency staff members can recommend certain counselors who are qualified to help someone with your specific issues.

Most public safety officers, EMS personnel, and health-care workers don't take their emotional well-being seriously enough. If you feel you need counseling, don't think that you're overreacting. Pick up the phone and get the ball rolling toward making this a reality.

In your initial sessions with a therapist, you will probably raise a lot of questions about the various areas of your life that are troubling you. This kind of cleansing of old emotional wounds can be painful. In fact, after a few initial sessions, you may become tempted to quit. Maybe talking about your problems seems like too much of a hassle. You don't like reflecting on them. Or, you can become tempted to halt the sessions because you're too busy.

Driving to the counselor's office every week will take a lot of effort. However, continue with the sessions not only for your own sake but also for the sake of your family and your career. Wait until both you and your counselor agree that you should stop.

Feeling in control won't happen overnight for anyone in counseling. In fact, in the beginning, almost everyone in counseling feels somewhat frustrated. It is natural to want quick relief. But it will take time for your therapist to help you unpack the heavy baggage you've been carrying around. As you lighten that load—by significantly reducing negative thoughts about painful issues—you should begin to feel better. The energy you've spent on coping with pain *can be reinvested back into your life*. You won't feel trapped and out of control anymore.

When your stress levels are critical, you should do everything necessary to gain support. For example, if you are single and living alone, you may want to sleep at a friend's house for a few nights. Or, you might decide to move back in with your parents for a month, depending on how they feel about it.

Reminder

Reach out for support in any way that feels right to you. Explain to others how they can help and why. For example, if you need to call an EMS chaplain twice a day, in addition to your counseling, explain to him or her: "I just need to hear a supportive person ask me how things are going."

Never feel embarrassed about reaching out for help. Until you feel more on top of things, find support in every way that makes sense to you. If you need to alternate spending time with your parents and a friend, that's fine. Being alone can be unbearable when you are severely depressed.

A natural approach can work

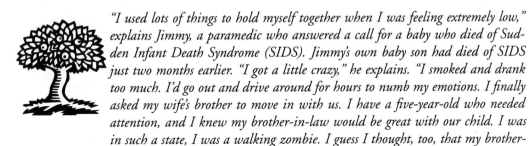

"I used lots of things to hold myself together when I was feeling extremely low," explains Jimmy, a paramedic who answered a call for a baby who died of Sudden Infant Death Syndrome (SIDS). Jimmy's own baby son had died of SIDS just two months earlier. "I got a little crazy," he explains. "I smoked and drank too much. I'd go out and drive around for hours to numb my emotions. I finally asked my wife's brother to move in with us. I have a five-year-old who needed attention, and I knew my brother-in-law would be great with our child. I was in such a state, I was a walking zombie. I guess I thought, too, that my brother-in-law would protect me if I thought about doing something crazy to myself."

Jimmy continues: *"Finally, I decided to get on a health kick. I felt better almost right away. I started taking vitamins, exercising, and eating better. I used herbal teas from the health food store to help me fall asleep. The nutritionist there recommended a couple of kinds which are known sleep enhancers. Sleep is so important. There's just no substitute for it, and these teas really helped make me drowsy. The bottom line about vitamins and natural substances, however, is that you don't want to bend the rules. They should be taken according to directions, because you can overuse anything."*

Like Jimmy, if you are under severe stress, you'll probably need all kinds of ways to comfort yourself. It can be tempting to use drugs and alcohol to ease the pain. However, coping this way will only prolong your getting well. Like Jimmy, you may find that natural remedies such as using herbal teas to help you sleep or taking vitamins will start you on the road to feeling better. Nurture yourself in ways that will benefit you over the long haul.

Try the following ways to soothe yourself when depression has escalated:

1. **Work something positive into each day.** This may be something as simple as talking with an upbeat person, watching a video you enjoy, or asking your spouse to give you a back rub. Deliberately focus on creating a positive experience each day, so that you can feel a measure of control over your day's outcome.

2. **Avoid negative people and negative conversations.** Go ahead and turn off the news if it's depressing. Steer away from depressing articles in the newspaper or turn off radio programs with negative themes.

3. **Get out in nature every single day, if possible.** If you don't have a beach or park near you, try walking in a nice neighborhood. Focus on the trees, shrubs, and flowering plants. Tune into things that grow because they are an affirmation of life itself.

4. **Do something to satisfy the child in you.** Stop at a ball field and watch a baseball game. Or play a few video games at the mall. Buy yourself an inexpensive toy. As an emergency responder, you've taken on an "adult" role of caretaking others. Sometimes, it is easy to forget that you still have a "child" within your psyche—the child you once were who is still a part of you. This child needs attention and care. As an adult, you can learn to "parent" this unique and sensitive part of yourself.

Remember that it always helps to have very clear-cut "coping goals." These goals can speed recovery, because they give you something to aim for. For instance, Betty, a young firefighter, was battling some terribly disturbing emotions after her partner was killed in a fire. "I blamed the building's owner for being too cheap to keep the wiring up to code," says Betty. "I blamed the city's inspectors, too. I was caught up in hate, but I didn't want to keep feeling that way."

Betty told herself, "I've been through a horrendous ordeal. But my partner was a person who did not harbor hate or bitterness. My goal in counseling and my recovery program is to work through this. I want to get to the point where I hate no one. I choose not to let hate overtake my thinking."

UNDERSTANDING ABUSE CALLS*

So how can you better serve others and yourself, when you are involved in scenes that involve true victims? How can you stay within your role in a domestic violence incident or a child abuse call? At some point in your career, you probably will have to answer at least one such call. A major stress factor for you will be this: How can you deal with your feelings concerning the perpetrator of the abuse? It is important to learn more about those who abuse in order to cope well.

Statistics reveal that child abuse incidents and domestic violence cases are increasing every year. Emergency dispatchers report they are receiving more and more calls for help, especially in larger cities. In child abuse incidents, these calls are often placed by injured children themselves. 911 dispatchers report that they sometimes hear a small voice coming over the line. Children as young as four years old have called to say: "My daddy's hitting me. Can you help?"

Attending a child who has been severely beaten, burned, or sexually assaulted can trigger many out-of-control emotions. Your own childhood experiences can also affect your reactions. For example, if you personally suffered any type of abuse as a child, you're likely to be more deeply affected than your coworkers. You might start to bond with the abused child, due to your feelings of wanting to protect him or her. Emotional flashbacks of your own abuse might become a problem also.

When your stress levels are already high, your involvement with a child abuse incident can be the last straw. You might become tempted to quit emergency work. In fact, lots of EMS personnel do throw in the towel and seek other career options after working a child abuse call.

Coping correctly will mean understanding your own feelings about abuse, educating yourself about why abuse happens, and appreciating the opportunity you have to help break a devastating cycle. The key to coping well is to concentrate on helping one child at a time. "Thinking about all the abused children out there will cripple you," says Vicky Byrd, past director of the Children's Advocacy Center in Sullivan County, Tennessee. "Focusing on one child at a time gives you the sense of control you need."

---

* Because many emergency responders choose to leave their respective professions after working a child abuse call, it is important to assess your thinking about such calls *before they arise,* if possible. Perhaps reading this section on how some professionals view child abuse will help you figure out ways to take more control of your emotions in various incidents involving violence. Emergency responders help to break a very destructive cycle of behavior by just being at the scene. You may be able to help more individuals, and hopefully deal more constructively with your own emotions, when you realize the value of your work in these trying episodes.

Byrd, who coordinated the emergency workers, hospital staff, social workers, and legal personnel assigned to help abused children in Sullivan County for several years, says, "Once the cycle of abuse is broken and family counseling begins, the child's life can begin to improve. There are some great success stories on record. *Emergency providers do help break the cycle.* From the moment they're dispatched to a scene, the child is no longer *alone* in handling the craziness."

Seeing a pediatric patient who has been hurt is never easy. Your emotional response will be the direct result of attitudes you have developed throughout life. You could easily be tempted to confront the abusive adult verbally or physically. In fact, some EMS providers have lost control at the scene. They've shoved, struck, or verbally attacked the suspected offender. In spite of the legal repercussions one could face, it is normal to feel a child deserves this show of support.

The best way to help the child, however, is to act calm and try to stay neutral and objective. This will take a lot of willpower, but your acting calm will help the child. A child in this situation hasn't begun to sort out his or her personal feelings. The child *does not* feel separated from the abuser's control just because you are at the scene.

From the moment you arrive at the scene, remember that the child's anxieties *will begin to escalate* because the family "secret" is now public knowledge. If you agitate the abuser in any way, you will add to the child's fear. He or she will worry that further punishment is coming to him or her. (The same feelings apply to an injured adult who has been abused in a domestic violence attack.)

> *"Controlling your emotions at the scene will mean you can stay alert and pay attention to details," says Connie, a first responder who testified in three child abuse trials and one domestic violence trial last year. "The more details you can provide legal authorities, the more credible you'll be as a witness if the abuser is prosecuted."*
>
> *Connie points out that another reason to stay calm is that self-blame can arise, if you can't recall information that might make a difference in court. "This is especially true if your patient is an injured child," says Connie.*

Vicky Byrd agrees. "You'll really need to keep your eyes and ears open in order to be an advocate for the child," she insists. "Those first at the scene should listen carefully to what the child says. Most children will say very little because they're terrified. It's important for emergency personnel to report what they saw and heard without second-guessing themselves."

It takes a broad team of legal, psychological, and medical experts to manage a single child abuse case. Each person doing his or her job thoroughly helps ensure the process works. As a medical provider, your job is to give care, furnish information to certain authorities, deal with stress, and then *emotionally distance yourself* from the case. "Otherwise, you won't survive," says Vicky Byrd.

You will probably feel physically and emotionally drained during the hours following a child abuse call or a domestic violence scene. It's exhausting to suppress strong emotions. There are specific ways to work through your feelings, but it may take days to even *begin* the process. Because you will be tempted to numb yourself psychologically, it might take time before you can identify your true feelings.

The emotional strain will be more complex if it is your first child abuse call or a particularly gruesome or violent incident. Your human values will be violated upon witnessing abuse of another individual. It's not unusual to feel some sort of personal connection to the devastation.

For instance, you may need to ask yourself why an incident is affecting you in a personal way. Does the abused child remind you of your own child? Did the nonabusive parent's passive attitude bother you? Does the abuser look like somebody you know?

Paul, a paramedic from the Northwest, couldn't work for days following a child abuse call. "I finally figured out the four-year old boy who'd been shoved off a balcony triggered feelings of guilt in me," he explains. "At that time, which was three years ago, I had a six-year-old son I wasn't spending enough time with. His mother and I are divorced, and I'd been neglecting him. After I worked the child abuse call, I moved across town to be closer to my son. This move was positive for everyone, so at least something good came from my stress."

Dealing with a child abuse call means you will wrestle with some of the most frustrating questions in our society. How could a mother hurt her own baby? What type of father injures a seven-year-old? Why would a mother passively allow her boyfriend to harm her child?

Understanding more about child abuse can help you cope. Child abuse is a complex subject, but having even a little knowledge about it can ease some of the confusion you might feel. Having no clue about why abuse occurs is one of the main stress factors for those who witness it.

Violence toward a child or anyone can be acted out suddenly—or over several hours or days. Violence is a mental explosion fueled by intense frustration. Individuals who abuse others have dozens, perhaps hundreds, of neglected emotional and physical needs. They carry frustrations that have increased daily since childhood. Abusers themselves have often explained their violent episodes to social workers and judges this way: "I start feeling pressure inside me. I'm like a tire that is blowing up. Then I explode."

Understanding loss of control

In order to understand how anyone could get to a violent state, try using your imagination for a moment. Picture what it would be like to endure a series of extremely stressful events. Let's say, for the sake of understanding, that you lost your job today. You leave work and drive home to find that your basement has flooded. To add insult to injury, your spouse is blaming you for not calling a plumber to fix the leak.

Let's say that you spend the next two hours sweeping water out of your basement. Then you decide to check your mailbox. It's full of overdue bills. The bills went unpaid because your child has been ill. You had to buy expensive prescriptions out of your paycheck. As you try to stay calm and tell yourself the world isn't coming to an end, the family dog jumps up and sharply bites your hand. What would you do to the dog?

However you'd choose to react—either by screaming at the dog or by inflicting physical punishment—your response would be largely determined by your *accumulated frustration.* The only reason you might not murder the dog would be because you would have to answer to your family and friends. Having a network of supportive people does trigger one's conscience, to be sure. But having a family and supportive friends also cushions the blows of life for you.

A child abuser or someone who would violently assault a spouse has compressed frustration in his psyche that would be difficult for most of us to imagine. Most likely, he or she was abused as a child. Throughout life, the abuser has never found emotional support that endured for any length of time. This person feels isolated from other people and can find no way to get relief from problems.

In a child abuse incident, a child with a difficult personality or an irritating cry can serve to trigger violence within the abuser. In addition, dozens of factors contribute to child abuse that have nothing to do with the child's behavior. For example, most abusive adults can't understand that children are dependent beings. In fact, they are so out of touch with their parental role, that they believe *a child should meet their needs in some way.*

Despite briefings about child abuse, it won't be easy to keep your cool at a scene where you have strong reasons to suspect a child has been physically violated. A mother may be screaming accusations at a boyfriend, or marks on a child's body may look suspicious.

"Emergency responders should remember that each incident must be carefully examined on its own merit," says Cleland Blake, M.D., a forensic pathologist in Morristown, Tennessee, who is an expert on abuse of children and the elderly. Dr. Blake, who has helped convict child abusers across the country in major trials, cautions: "Most child abuse cases are legitimate, but people do make false charges occasionally. Parents sometimes want to get revenge on an ex-spouse or a lover."

He continues, "I've witnessed a few rare cases in which a child has lied about the abuse. For example, I once medically examined three preteen girls who claimed a male relative had sexually molested them. For reasons of their own, these children had invented their story. They had not been molested."

Emergency personnel who have worked child abuse calls experience the whole gamut of negative emotions such as disbelief, fear, intense rage, and guilt about neglected people in our society. Some may suffer self-blame if the call was a repeat call to the *same address.*

"The question that haunted me was: 'Why couldn't I have done something ear-lier to stop this?'" says Barbara, paramedic supervisor who has worked three such incidents in her home state of Florida over the past several years. "In each of the cases I worked, I was called back a number of times to one address and twice to the other two. Parents who abuse become expert liars. Social workers are overloaded with cases. The police don't know what to do, and neither do we. Anger and feelings of helplessness are the two most intense emotions emergency responders must deal with after a child abuse call."

These three self-help measures can put you more in control during the first few days when you're not sure how to cope:

- **Vent your anger by writing your thoughts down.** One New Jersey EMT worked a child abuse call in which a father had shaken the baby so violently that death resulted. "Writing my thoughts down helped me vent without driving my coworkers up the wall," he says. "My wife had recently suffered a miscarriage, and here was a father who'd killed his own baby. By pouring out my thoughts and feelings on paper I was able to release a lot of anger."

- **Don't condemn all of society.** Don't allow yourself to think, "The world has gone to hell." Thinking like this diminishes all hope about your own future. Of course, it is normal in the beginning to think, "I'd like to strangle that abusive father with my own two hands." Even social workers, counselors, and doctors react this way. It is vital to focus on the good things in society when you've met with an act of violence.

- **Take positive action.** Although talking out feelings with a psychologist, coworker, or spouse certainly helps, you might still feel powerless. Your talking things out, after all, isn't helping the injured child. A realistic plan of action can help offset this lack of power. Implementing some kind of positive action on behalf of the injured child will pump some of your adrenaline into helping society at large.

Tony, a paramedic from New York State, says, "I was frustrated about a child abuse call I'd worked. The doctor acted unsure about the abuse. It looked as if the mother's boyfriend was going to get off the hook. I was livid. My own father had abused me, and I couldn't stand this injustice."

He continues, "My wife told me to do something positive. She reminded me I could do something to help other abused children. I asked a social worker to hold a seminar on child abuse at four of our local schools. This might not sound like much, but I did feel better. Spending some energy on making a tiny difference is better than feeling totally helpless to change anything."

Though a child abuse incident is not something to trivialize, it helps to stay focused on positive outcomes that result from it. For example, news coverage starts a snowball effect. Usually a dozen other child abuse incidents are reported to authorities when one case gets media attention.

LOOK AT THE HOPEFUL SIDE

Before you get any more depressed, try to stay calm and gather the facts. The situation may not be as hopeless as it looks—even if the child is still living in the home.

"Not every child abuser is a monster or a psychotic," says John Stringer, a social worker with the Washington County Human Services Department in Bristol, Virginia. "The paramedic only gets the ugly picture at the scene. Social workers, however, treat child abuse as a family problem. Often the stress is just temporary, especially if there's no money or food in the house."

He continues, "Keep in mind that a child-abuse case is never as cut and dried as it looks. For example, it may turn out that the parent doing the blaming was actually the one doing the hitting. This may come out in family interaction with a social worker or at any step during the investigation."

A doctor's examination can determine extensive abuse or clear-cut abuse over a period of time. But there are plenty of borderline cases in which the facts aren't clear. Did the child get a black eye by wrecking a bike? Or did the child's father inflict it? In some of these cases, the parent really is innocent.

When you are involved in a confusing case, gaining more information will help you feel more in control.

Follow these guidelines for finding out more:

- **Visit the social worker in charge of the case.** Although details are confidential, you can find out the agency's procedure for helping families in such a situation. In most states, those who report child abuse have some rights to information by law. If you get nowhere with the social worker, ask to see the agency's supervisor, who can tell you in very general terms what the system can or cannot do.

- **Get information about your county's processing guidelines.** Learn about all the steps that are taken in every reported case. Just hearing how much effort goes into fact checking, both medically and legally, may help you feel better.

- **Call the child's school psychologist.** Never, under any circumstances, identify yourself or the child. But do find out if an education program on abuse has been implemented. Are teachers well instructed on how to spot abuse and report it? Are hotline numbers clearly posted where children can see them?

Sometimes, however, child abuse incidents you work may involve children under school age or infants. They might not have the same advantages as a child in school for obtaining help. These children are much more vulnerable. How can you deal psychologically with these kinds of fears?

Although you must accept that you are limited in what you can do, you don't have to take a purely negative approach. Professionals who deal with child abuse offer these guidelines for feeling hopeful:

- **People are much more willing to report abuse than they were a decade ago.** Neighbors, health-care workers, and relatives are coming forward more readily. Why? Laws of confidentiality, coupled with education efforts, have made people more responsible about picking up the phone. As a result of early reporting, blatant physical and sexual abuse of children can be more easily documented.

- **Remember that things do change.** A mother's boyfriend may leave for good, a grandmother may move into the home to offer assistance, or a new job can ease the family's stress.

- **Sometimes it takes a second effort.** When the system fails the first time around, relatives or neighbors may file another complaint right away. A child abuse case can be reopened at any time.

- **It is usually best to keep a child with his or her family.** Although this is not true for criminal or sexual abuse, it is true in cases where families are receptive to help offered—as many families are. Emotional counseling and financial help can make a big difference in the home's atmosphere.

- **Know the limits of your own profession.** As an EMT, police officer, or volunteer firefighter, you are only one link in the chain of help for a child. Be very firm with yourself in knowing what your job entails. It is virtually impossible for you to do any other professional's job in the system. Focus on your own role and do it well. Find a cutoff point where you can say, "I've done everything possible to help this individual child."

Obtaining a point of closure doesn't mean that you can't check in with the child's case three to six months from now. In addition, for your own peace of mind, you always have the option of driving by the house to see the child playing outside.

When you keep your emotions in check, you can spend your mental energy in a very productive way. This is key to preventing burnout. Focus your attention on helping the next child who might need help in coping with abuse.

Make each case a learning experience. Remember that no experience goes to waste if you take time to assess it properly. Some small detail you learn in a chaotic incident of violence could help you in a nonabusive situation with another child. Or, you might pick up a clue that could help you identify an abusive situation with a geriatric patient. A good emergency responder is also very much an investigator. By learning to enjoy this learning opportunity, you can help to prevent burnout.

Dr. Cleland Blake has this attitude of positive focus in his forensic work: "With abused individuals I do focus on what's going to make a difference," he asserts. "I've been able to help a lot of abused people by not giving in to negative thinking. A lot of doctors refuse to examine or help abused patients because of the legal red tape and time they'd spend in court. I focus on the unique opportunity I have to go to bat for these people."

As an EMT, paramedic, rescue worker, or firefighter, you might feel you can't really make a substantial difference in helping an abused child. But child abuse specialists like Dr. Blake feel emergency providers *will be heroes the child remembers throughout life.* Your calm and objective attitude and how you handle the situation overall will contribute greatly to the child's well being.

Further tips for coping with calls involving violence:

- **Take it one step at a time.** When you're interviewed by social workers or legal personnel, focus on answering one question at a time about the incident.

- **Give your best answers and never second-guess yourself.** Don't create stress in yourself by lying awake nights wondering if your answers were good enough.

- **Watch how you deal with the public.** When people approach you in the supermarket to inquire, "Did that sick monster really do those things to that little girl?" you may be tempted to talk too much. You're only human, and it can feel good to get some things off your chest. But stick with neutral remarks such as, "Child abusers were probably abused themselves."

Remember that your involvement in a scene involving violence is a legal issue. If you share confidential information, it may come back to haunt you. Juan, a first responder who helped with a sexual abuse incident in the late 1980s, says: "I was new at my job, and I didn't realize sex offenders, until convicted, have the same legal rights as anyone. I talked too much to people about it, and they furnished details around town. Naturally, they attached my name to their stories. If my boss had gotten wind of it, I would have been fired."

Child abuse isn't going to end tomorrow, but you can do small things to help curtail some of it. For example, you might encourage your emergency division to organize a community education program on child abuse. Your fire station or EMS unit could arrange for experts on child abuse to speak at schools and churches. Children can be taught how to find help if they need it.

It is a myth that all teachers and doctors will find and report abuse. Most adults will sidestep child abuse issues because they don't want to get involved. They may not want to spend the time or effort in helping, or they may be afraid they are sounding a false alarm.

Being an advocate of good child-care programs that are affordable to poor or single-parent households is also taking a stand against child abuse. "A mother who's forced to use her boyfriend as a baby sitter while she works is one of the most dangerous situations in our society," says Dr. Cleland Blake. "That boyfriend will resent those children. He will likely abuse them verbally or physically."

Educating yourself about child abuse, what you can do about it, and how to deal with your emotions linked to personal involvement with it will take a period of time. You can't do it in a few days. A child abuse call you have worked might have a long term impact on you no matter how well you handle it.

Try to examine your feelings openly until you can talk about them in a very forthright and objective way. In a very real sense, this type of processing helps to transfer painful emotions to the more logical areas of your brain. Having this objectivity helps you to appropriately *respond* to what has happened, rather that just *react* to it. Your feelings are an important part of you, and you're entitled to "own" them, regardless of how someone else would handle the same situation. However, if you can examine your thoughts and feelings from a calmer, more logical state of mind, you can obtain a mental "closure" much more successfully. You can close the book and move past the painful event.

CRITICAL INCIDENT STRESS MANAGEMENT

As an emergency responder, you will deal with a lot of medical problems and injuries. But there is also a good chance you will face surprises by Mother Nature in your career. Earthquakes, floods, hurricanes, tornadoes, wildfires, and other natural disasters can arise. Tragedies such as explosions or acts by terrorists can occur also. Your own stress can become very complex and unmanageable as you watch survivors face the aftermath. It can be excruciatingly painful to watch others deal with loss of loved ones, their homes, and their possessions.

In the early 1980s, a disturbing trend was emerging from the ranks of EMS workers. Many were becoming victims themselves as they struggled to protect and save others. The psychological pain they were experiencing is now called *critical incident stress*. Today there are sophisticated ways of dealing with this trauma through *critical incident stress management (CISM)* programs.

Dr. Jeffrey Mitchell, of Baltimore, Maryland, created the first critical incident stress management program. Critical incident stress is any situation faced by emergency services personnel that causes them to experience unusually strong emotional reactions. These reactions have the potential to interfere with their ability to cope at the scene or afterward.

> *"For months after I worked an earthquake incident, I'd sit up in bed shaking from fear," says Delores, a first responder. "I had a particularly bad dream that kept recurring. I wanted to block it out of my mind, but you can't control your dreams. I think that Critical Incident Stress Debriefing would have helped me, if I'd participated. But after the earthquake, I took a leave of absence. I had a lot of feelings I should have discussed with my coworkers, but to tell you the truth, I would have been afraid of sharing my thoughts and feelings openly at that time. I kind of ran away from EMS for about three years."*

When you participate in a CISD session, you learn that you are a normal person who is having normal responses to an abnormal situation. Because you are a kind and caring individual, you will react more strongly than someone who has less sensitive emotions. You are human, regardless of your training or your coping skills. Serious events can and do pierce the psyche of emergency responders. These events are so powerful that they override one's usual ability to cope.

What Is Critical Incident Stress Management?

CISM focuses on crisis intervention techniques. Those individuals trained to help you can offer tools for how you should share your stress *appropriately*. Sometimes, it feels better to share in a very low-key way. Or, you may need to talk about part of the incident in depth. Certain questions may keep coming into your mind. If you can share these questions openly, some of your colleagues may be able to offer insight. Those in charge of a debriefing will help you obtain the information you need. This knowledge will help you to establish a sense of closure.

When you are at a very stressful scene, your mind will tend to block out part of the pain in order to protect you. Someone else might have grasped something you didn't perceive or understand in the midst of the traumatic event. Every person at the scene will experience and interpret what happened in a unique way. In a *Critical Incident Stress Debriefing (CISD)*, you can reach out to others for support and clarification of what happened. Even if you feel no need to obtain more information, you may be able to help someone else at a debriefing session. Never underestimate how your sharing one small piece of information can help a fellow worker or individual affected by the trauma.

Unanswered questions can make anyone feel out of control. For example, feeling overwhelmed that you couldn't be more productive in helping others at a scene can cause you to feel inadequate, even guilty. Of course, gruesome scenes and harmful effects upon one's fellow man will affect any normal, sane, individual in an adverse way. CISD will help you to figure out what is significant about the work you were able to accomplish. The meetings will also help you to figure out which parts are better put to rest.

Your goal is to find a safe and comfortable way to deal with your thoughts and reactions. Without enough closure, your emotional wounds can't begin to heal properly. If you don't attend a CISD session, you may never find important answers you need to obtain closure. This is partly due to the fact that your colleagues will forget much of what happened if the debriefing session isn't held right away.

If possible, the session should be held within 72 hours after an incident. As time goes by, the facts about what transpired will become less clear .

The desired outcome of CISM is to return those experiencing traumatic stress to their normal, productive lives. Part of the CISM process involves working with the *healing power of group sessions.* For those who open up and fully participate, there is a bonding experience in a debriefing session. Being able to feel that others understand your pain is comforting.

> *Everyone affected by a traumatic incident or tragedy is invited to participate in a Critical Incident Stress Debriefing. However, many who are required to attend can resent it. "I've had employees act very upset about having to participate in a CISD session," says Leslie, director of an urban EMS division in the West. "My employees and I have often assisted in helping to clean up the aftermath of an earthquake or flood. Most of us are in bad shape psychologically after one of these events. But I always have a few people who protest the whole idea of a group debriefing. When I ask them more about their feelings, they act unsure about why they feel that way. A few responders even appear angry in these CISD meetings."*

Some individuals do not feel comfortable sharing pain in a group setting because of their past conditioning. For instance, they might have been raised in a family where open displays of emotions were frowned upon. In some families, one's being overly emotional is perceived as a weakness. So perhaps CISD should always be optional for emergency responders.

Much debate about the benefits of CISD is still going on, but the majority of responders seem to feel it is a wonderful forum for healing. When help is given soon after a traumatic event, individuals and communities can regain their peace of mind and wholeness, and EMS workers are able to continue with their important work.

Additionally, victims of critical incident stress may suffer from a potentially debilitating condition known as *Post Traumatic Stress Disorder (PTSD)*. This is similar to the same type of response combat veterans have in the military after a trying incident or period of extreme stress. Flashbacks of a particular scene can happen frequently, along with nightmares and a host of emotional and physical problems. Feelings of shock, fear, grief, emotional numbness, and helplessness are common. Memory loss and changes in how you feel about your family and friends can result, also. Relationships become difficult because PTSD can leave you feeling very disoriented and disconnected from others. Critical Incident Stress Debriefing after a stressful event *can help to prevent* this disorder.

Dealing with extreme job stress is never easy. However, if you take as many control measures as you can *early on,* you can help yourself manage the impact much more successfully. If you need to see a counselor, talk with a peer supporter, participate in a debriefing session, or figure out self-help measures, it is important to begin as soon as possible. Extreme stress is not good for the body or the brain.

Although self-help is always important, severe stress almost always requires that you reach out to others to assist you. Never hesitate to call a professional therapist or a mental health agency right away if you feel you need to. When you take responsibility for finding help, you will soon feel less vulnerable. After all, reaching out for help *is* a way of taking control in a bad situation. Your community, which you have served as an emergency responder, can provide the help you need.

REVIEW ACTIVITIES

1. Name two ways you could help yourself avoid negative thinking in a very stressful situation.

2. Why is it important to find an "authority figure" willing to listen to extremely stressful problems?

3. Why is it best to find out the names of excellent counselors before you get in a crisis situation?

4. Name two ways that counseling can help you deal with problems.

5. Why will talking too much about your problems make you feel worse?

6. Instead of reacting emotionally to a stressful situation, describe one way you might respond more logically in order to reduce your personal stress.

7. Describe why intense frustration causes those who abuse to explode and become violent.

8. Why would your calmness at a scene help a child or adult who has been abused feel less threatened?

9. How might Critical Incident Stress Debriefing sessions help you obtain closure after a traumatic incident?

FOR SUPERVISORS

1. One of your employees has confided that he or she is extremely depressed. You know that this employee has worked several intense calls recently. What plan of action would you encourage this person to take? How would you approach the idea of private counseling with this individual?

2. You are having recurring nightmares about one of your calls. Would you confide in your coworkers, or would you be worried that you could be perceived as weak? If you proceeded to receive private counseling, how would you feel about sharing this information with your employees and volunteers?

CLASS PROJECTS

1. Invite an EMS chaplain to speak to your class. Ask him or her to address the following topic: How can an individual actively listen and offer sensitive feedback to a coworker who is under extreme stress?

2. Ask members of a Critical Incident Stress Debriefing team to speak to the class about what they have learned in helping responders. For example, ask if they would be willing to share information about what to expect in a debriefing session. Perhaps they would share their personal viewpoints on helpful techniques in working with someone under extreme stress.

CHAPTER FIVE

LEADERS UNDER STRESS

"I *was sitting in a sports bar a couple of years ago," says Mike, a paramedic from New England. "I was celebrating the fact that my coworkers had elected me captain of our volunteer organization. Now, I'm sure they didn't worry about my qualifications. Somebody just threw my name in the hat.*

"Anyway, I was sipping a drink and watching a close hockey match on the bar's wide-screen TV, when two of my fellow medics came running into the place. 'Mike!' one of them called out, 'Some of our crew turned over an ambulance at the hospital entrance—you know, where that curve is so tricky. The police want to talk to you about our insurance.' His sidekick chimed in, 'The patient on board was a city official. I hope you don't mind that I gave the TV news people your pager number. I told them you'd be happy to talk with them on the six o'clock news.'"

Mike laughs now about how nervous he was on the news that day. "I remember thinking, 'I'm in over my head. I'm gonna kill those guys for electing me.'"

Whenever you accept a position of leadership, you need a certain set of skills to carry out your responsibilities. Like Mike, you'll no doubt have days when you're certain you have bitten off more than you can chew. But if you have a good attitude and are eager to learn, it can be exciting to find out how much you can accomplish. In fact, Mike went on to become an EMS consultant to his state legislators who were reviewing a bill concerning prehospital medical care.

Whether you are a manager in emergency response, or you run a chain of department stores, becoming a leader in today's world calls for having a complex set of skills. Not only must you manage yourself and your own personal set of stress factors, but you've got to acquire the expertise it takes to manage the actions of others.

You need to have people skills, public relations skills, and a measure of business–financial savvy. It is wise to educate yourself outside of the formal classroom continually. Competition in the workplace demands that everyone who wants to advance should be attending seminars, reading up on how to manage employees, and striving to implement new ideas into each workday. It even helps to be somewhat of an amateur psychologist. When you understand more about human behavior, you can better anticipate the needs and reactions of others.

Attaining more knowledge is imperative for taking charge of others, but how you *present yourself* to others is also vitally important in any leadership role. You always want to appear in control of yourself and your work environment. Without seeming pompous or egotistical, you need to create an aura around you that says, "I can be depended upon to lead."

To assess your present leadership skills, you will need to ask yourself probing questions such as these:

- **Do I come across as a disciplined person who cares about the job?** Leaders who set an example for excellence will solicit more respect. Are you self-directed, goal oriented, and meticulous about details? If you do just enough work to get by, your subordinates will do likewise.

  When it comes to being a caring type of leader, maybe you find this concept outmoded. Perhaps you've grown a little cynical, even tough, in order to cope. That's easy to do. But ideally, you want to care about your work and your coworkers. If you don't really care about anything except collecting your paycheck, your staff will pick up on this quickly. It will be hard for them to trust you.

- **Do I create a positive feeling around me?** All of us want to be led by strong, bold, optimistic people. Have you noticed how *draining* it is to be around a negative person who continually finds fault with the world? As a manager, you don't have to be a born cheerleader. But it helps to give off energetic "vibes" that tell others "I have a can-do attitude."

- **Am I empowering those around me?** Good leaders can visualize their own career path and the career paths of others. They enable and encourage others to make good choices. In addition, good leaders continually sharpen their delegation skills.

  The process of good delegating within your unit will strengthen your team. Many leaders grow weak and fail to advance themselves, because they try to *do* everything themselves. They fail to find and utilize the intelligence and talents of those under their supervision.

  "I used to be afraid of the delegating process," says Maria, now a captain in a mid-size fire–EMS department. "I was a control freak, because I'd learned early in life that other people can let you down. It took me a long time to get over this fear. I had a great mentor who explained to me: 'Maria, if you don't learn to

delegate you're really not being fair to your coworkers. You need to stop hogging the power.'"

Reminder

Those managers who fail to delegate skillfully and develop good employees will be blown away by the competition, especially if they are in private EMS. Wise leaders today know that employees are a department's most precious resource. Managers who act differently will be the downfall of their departments. Bringing out the best in others is the hallmark of a good leader.

You might believe that your private ambulance service, which has been in business for 25 years, is doing just fine. But if you fail to stretch the skills of your staff by continually delegating in the right way, there will come a time when your company will be far behind collectively on computer skills, community relations skills, and financial knowledge of EMS. It may be impossible to catch up.

A New Path Ahead

Leadership in the year 2000 and beyond will be very different than it was even 10 years ago. Leaders today cannot be truly effective by being arrogant or demanding. Nice guy tactics are very much the way to go. Employees respect leaders who are fair, honest, and consistent. They resent those in charge who are overly hard-nosed. Be-

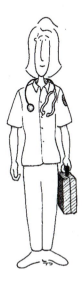

sides, anyone who is too pushy or demanding in the workplace setting needs more education in some area. A person acting aggressively, rather than assertively, shows that his or her communication skills and people skills need updating.

As a top-notch leader in EMS today, you have to think of yourself as someone who needs the business tools and management skills of a corporate CEO. You can't learn everything in a month or a year. But by reading good EMS journals, general business magazines, and attending educational conferences, you will be more inspired to try innovative ideas. Trying new things will help you to prevent career burnout, too.

Giving of yourself

Those in supervisory roles and managerial positions must think of themselves as a servant of people. Leaders who don't serve the needs of those on their team will forfeit power in the long run. For example, have you ever voted for a politician who got elected and then tried to "phone in" the required work? He or she didn't stay in touch with voters and their needs. It probably wasn't long until this politician had lost everyone's confidence.

Long gone are the days when bosses could worry solely about the financial bottom line and ignore the emotional and physical needs of their staff. For one thing, people are costly to train—and therefore costly to replace—if they decide to go elsewhere. But we're also living in a world where people need to bond at work in order to create surrogate families and meaningful networks. Everyone benefits when managers and leaders create an emotional bond of goodwill among their workers.

Sometimes, creating this bond is difficult to do. No one says that bringing about harmony in a department is a snap. This can be due to personality differences or any number of complex issues. For example, the political game of the moment might be rocking the company boat. But supervisors and managers who try hard to enhance team spirit are going to have less stress and a more productive division over the long haul.

Collin, an EMS supervisor in a large county department, shares this story: "I used to work in private EMS. For months, my boss had promised several people in our department a raise. Well, it was down to the deadline. Six medics were threatening to quit if no raise materialized. It didn't and they did quit."

He continues, "Our department's morale sank like the Titanic *that day. My boss, who was the owner of the company, wanted me to get busy and raise the* Titanic. *He instructed me to share with our remaining employees lots of details about our department's needs. Well, I did as I was told, but I felt like the lowest human on the planet. It was like insulting the crew on a sinking ship by talking about the needs of the ship's owner. If I had it to do over, I would have handled it differently. I would have worked on my approach. How a leader conveys information can be destructive or supportive. That company is still in business, but employee turnover is high. The owner's attitude hasn't changed a bit."*

Tom Hornsby, a speaker and writer on work-related issues who lives in Kingsport, Tennessee, believes that political games in the work setting will become less intense when leaders demonstrate true support to employees in every way they can. He encourages everyone in the workplace setting to think about *why* they need to care about those in their circle of influence. He calls this concept "the big world theory." Hornsby points out that most of us believe we live in a very large global community. However, he emphasizes that it is quite the contrary.

"Let's say that you know two hundred and fifty people or more on a first-name basis," Hornsby explains. "In fact, you might know a thousand people. But still, this is not a lot of people. If you know just these few people, out of billions on the planet, then why would you want to play games? Why would you want to do anything except be a good person to those you know?'

He continues, "Leaders must become coaches, instead of control supervisors. Leadership must care about people and show it."

Reminder

As a leader, you set the tone for the troops. Your beliefs and attitudes will rub off on everyone around you. Coaching others to do their best can be perceived as stressful or as challenging. It all depends upon the attitude of the coach. It certainly is your job to help employees deal constructively with their weaknesses. But find their strengths early on, too. *It's the collective strengths of employees that will run your organization.*

When employees have an outlet for sharing their strengths, they won't be as likely to act out their needs for recognition via destructive politics. After all, political games acted out in any profession can be just a way of saying, "I'm going to make sure I find some control—even if I have to scheme and manipulate!" When workers are focused on making a solid contribution, and their self-esteem is high, political games tend to fall by the wayside.

COACHING WELL

Being a "talent coordinator" is what good leadership is about. To find out the talents of individuals, you've got to pay close attention. You need to have private conversations with employees in order to evaluate them as individuals. It can also be beneficial to ask them to assess each other's strengths. Remind individuals to *carefully assess their own weaknesses.* It is certainly no fun for any of us to have someone else point out our flaws. Encourage those you supervise to devise a plan for overcoming any weaknesses and turning them into strengths. For example, each employee might write a simple plan for improving three skills over the next four months.

If you have an employee who needs education in a certain area, it can be productive to put that individual in charge of researching what he or she needs to know. Then have that person teach this information to others.

> *William, a veteran administrator in the fire services, shares this story about how he got a misinformed employee moving in the right direction: "I hired a young man who was an excellent firefighter/paramedic. The only problem was, he loved to make 'complimentary remarks' to our female employees. He didn't mean any harm. But this was the era when people were beginning to sue employers and coworkers on sexual harassment charges. He needed to rethink his ideas on how to treat women."*

> *William continues, "I called this young man aside and explained to him that I needed his help. I told him, 'I know you love reading and research, because you've presented some excellent materials in training sessions. I've got an area to address that is a very sensitive issue. I wondered if you'd be willing to read up on what's appropriate behavior for males and females toward each other in the work setting?'*

> *"He was happy to comply. He went to a lot of trouble to find good information. I got so tickled watching him present this material—and so did everyone else. He was a good sport, and he did clean up his own act toward the women in our department. He even put up news clippings on our bulletin board about the details of sexual harassment cases."*

In order to lower your own stress levels as a leader, remind yourself that you are a coordinator of talents. Remember that you are not qualified to fix personality problems. For your own sake, don't try to remedy too many petty problems, either. Pick important battles and important issues to address. It is not your job to referee childish quarrels or to listen to an overabundance of personal problems. It also is not your place to make your employees like each other. It is your job to build a structure of talents and skills within your organization.

By working to create the path to get your division to where it needs to be, you won't spend all of your time reacting to things. Going into a more creative mode can boost your effectiveness when you're in charge. Here's why:

- **Visualizing creates the road map you need.** For example, if you need to get your organization from full-time firefighting to firefighting and EMS, you need to spend time picturing how to bring this about. For example, which phone calls should you make first? What materials from your state health department would be beneficial? How can you take your division from point A to point B without wasting steps?

- **Affirmations create determination.** Whether you write down sentences that affirm positive thoughts—or say them a few times over to yourself on the way to work—they can instill a sense of focus in you.

  You shouldn't waste time affirming near-impossibilities such as: "I'll find a way to double everyone's salary by next year." But good, reasonable affirmations keep you fixated on success. For example, by repeating to yourself, "I'll find three good ways to motivate my people this quarter," you are setting a goal that's doable.

- **Remember to coach yourself constantly.** Leaders must talk to themselves a lot. Usually the communication is silent. But what we tell ourselves each day does make a difference in what we accomplish and what we get others to do. Positive self-talk helps keep any leader centered and more relaxed so he or she can have more productive days.

It always helps to use self-talk that steers you to specific, positive action. For example, if you have a gigantic problem staring you in the face, try telling yourself, "I'll tackle the impossible by breaking it down into tiny steps. Maybe I can't make a lot of progress on this immediately, but I'll begin by doing something small. At least I'll get the wheels turning."

Keep your self-talk geared to encouraging yourself when stress is mounting and you feel you're getting snowed under. For example, by telling yourself, "I'm proud of the way I handled my workload this week," you are being supportive of yourself. Don't increase your stress by indulging in self-doubt and self-recrimination when things aren't going well. You'll only break down your own morale.

Some tactics that can help you have more fun with your leadership role are these:

- **Learn to ask more intelligent questions.** If you learn to ask better questions, you will get better answers. For example, if two of your employees can't get along, you could ask yourself, "How can I get these blockheads to stop quarreling?" A more intelligent and productive question might be "How can I help these two see more of each other's viewpoint?"

- **Practice asking "how" instead of "why."** For example, if your department's budget is a disaster, you could spend all day asking "Why did we let ourselves get into this mess?" But when you start asking *"How* can we find a new approach?" or *"How* can I find expert advice on fixing this?" or *"How* can we tackle this issue aggressively and win?" you'll be empowering yourself. Keep asking "how" questions until solutions start to emerge.

- **Do something each day that will make a difference a year from now.**
Making a slight improvement in scheduling, contacting an interesting
speaker for a training session, or praising an EMT in front of his or her
fellow workers are small acts that can have big payoffs later.

If worse comes to worst

In most instances, your employees do have a choice in how they will respond to your
leadership efforts. For example, some will always choose to do the minimum to get
by. Or, some will choose to be unreceptive to positive mentoring. You can't win
every time, regardless of your good intentions. Your goal should be to do your best
while creating *the least stress for yourself.*

When a crisis occurs, focus on what is going to help your department. Even if
a major problem arises—such as several employees quitting in one day—remind
yourself that you can regain control. You can do that if you resolve to work *with people,* not against them. For example, when employees make it clear they have lost
faith in management, you can't necessarily fix their opinions. But you can let them
share their concerns very openly and still let them know *that you are very much in
control.*

*Try these suggestions when a depressing situation has
materialized within your department:*

- **Use honesty to help everyone feel grounded.** If a situation is bad, admit it. The worst thing you can do is to downplay it. Identify what has
gone wrong and let everyone speak about the situation either in an
open forum or in a private meeting with you. Tell those under your supervision: "I want you to express your feelings. Don't attack anyone personally, but do express how this situation is affecting you."
- **Set a time limit allowed for complaints.** You might say, "Let's talk
about this very openly for the next 45 minutes. I want you to get everything off your chest, and I promise I will listen closely to what you have
to say."

  You need to define how long you are willing to hear complaints,
because you don't want these complaints lasting for six months. Try to
help everyone see that it is to their benefit to speak up honestly to clear
the air and then let the issue go. Then tell them, "If you need to discuss
this in private outside of work, that's fine. I understand that this is
painful for you. But I must require that we end the discussion on this
here at the station."

- **After the smoke has cleared, insist that everyone get a new focus.** Ask each person, "What talents and skills do you have to offer this department? I'm sorry that we have a negative situation going on, but we have to start fresh. We have to rebuild our unit, and I want each of you to share how you plan to help."

By helping workers focus on what they have to give, you'll be assuming your rightful role—leading the troops away from defeatism. By requiring them to focus on themselves and their skills, you are helping them to feel a sense of rededication to the department. You might choose to have everyone share his or her strengths openly with you. Consider asking each person to write a personal mission statement to share with you. It all depends on your management style.

Although you don't have to act as if several workers quitting is nothing—and you'd be foolish to take such a crisis casually—you don't want to lose control of the reins. Turning everyone's attention toward his or her own sense of worth says: "I'm rebuilding the team—better and stronger."

Doubting Thomases

"Well, this all sounds good in theory," you might say, "but you don't know how bad it is for me. Nice guy tactics won't work on the people I deal with! They have more ego and personality problems than you can shake a stick at."

Although personality problems, family problems, and intense work stress can cause employees to be uncooperative and moody, you can still find ways to feel in control of your department. It won't happen overnight, but it can happen if you start by *changing yourself*. When you change yourself, everyone around you is encouraged to change. By taking responsibility for improving your leadership skills, you are sending this message to employees: "I want to raise the standards for myself and all of you."

One way to bring out the best in everyone is to make sure there is a career success track for each employee. This will require that you give personal attention to each employee. Helping individuals to set goals and keep track of any progress is always a productive way to motivate others. Of course, all employees can't be promoted at once. Nor can everyone always get a raise in pay every quarter. However, it is easier for an individual to work within a department if leaders help him or her to make a productive contribution.

The day-to-day work of that individual should be monitored for needed feedback, whenever possible. Plus, supervisors should be helpful in giving out "growth assignments" via the delegation process. Supervisors should also be on the lookout

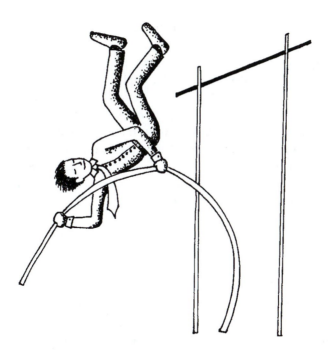

for employee efforts that deserve praise. Working with each person's talents will help prevent the onset of ugly politics and unproductive competitiveness.

This is not to say that you, as a manager or leader, won't have to play any political games yourself at work. Everyone does to some degree. There are times when you'll have to patronize your immediate boss or even community leaders. Sometimes, you'll have to avoid confrontations skillfully. There will be occasions when you probably will be dragged into a few discussions you would rather avoid—as you try to stay tightlipped.

Conversely, there are times when you *must* throw a piece of information into the company "gossip pool." After all, if the grapevine closes down to you, you'll be out on a limb by yourself. The best leaders and employees have to play politics to a certain degree. Good leaders will concentrate on building teamwork, helping others grow, and working to find common ground, activities which enhance the pride of everyone in the department.

We all like to work with those people with easygoing, pleasant personalities who can get along with everyone. But often that's not the case. Almost everyone has to work with a few people they don't especially like. Savvy supervisors learn to get the "good" out of people. You don't want to manipulate people in a selfish way, but you do need to manipulate *situations* whereby every person in your department can make the *best contribution*. It is called helping others to succeed. *This approach helps everyone and hurts no one.*

THE FINE ART OF DELEGATION

Giving out certain tasks or assignments can make any supervisor uneasy. What if an employee or volunteer flubbed the responsibility—maybe costing your department lots of time or money. Or, what if a project you give away is handled really well—so well that it impresses top management. You might worry that those under you will do a *better job* than you could have. Who needs the competition?

Though handing power over to others can be uncomfortable, it is not as self-defeating nor as risky as it seems. Good delegating will enhance your ability to develop a team of people. Plus, when you spread the work around, you will be freer to tackle bigger assignments yourself.

You can't just manage people anymore. In today's world of EMS, fire, and law enforcement work, you have to think in terms of leading people toward goals. Good leaders move people toward greater goals by slowly stretching them to assume more responsibility.

How much to delegate and what to delegate has to be based on the training and experience of employees. However, good delegators keep their eyes on "stretch" projects for workers. These projects will take a well-trained individual a little beyond what he or she is used to. This helps develop that person step-by-step. This stretching should be an ongoing process that gradually takes everybody to the next level of responsibility.

Because emergency work involves so much stress from working calls, you can help your personnel manage the stress by encouraging everyone to diversify his or her workday. All employees should be involved in business matters, employees' training needs, and general improvements for the department.

People feel more satisfied with their jobs when they are asked for creative input. Delegating effectively helps employees contribute to the big picture. It helps them feel valued. Money isn't everything. People in emergency work want more than money. Enabling them to carry out interesting assignments helps motivate them to try more.

Reminder

Whenever possible, it is good to give people total control to make decisions. If a committee is in charge, let the group develop its own strategies. Figuring out a plan of action in a group helps coworkers bond with each other. Also, a supervisor's faith in their decisions helps them feel empowered to lead.

EMS and firefighting units in larger cities often use the team concept in delegating the workload. It is common for them to have employment committees that review applicants, reprimand committees that discipline their peers, vehicle and equipment committees that recommend purchases, and quality assurance committees that review performance details of emergency calls.

When you delegate work to a committee, it is a good idea to choose people for the group who have diverse talents. For example, let's say you have created a vehicle committee that will solicit bids for new ambulances. You might place someone on the committee who has a financial background, another with good clerical skills, one with grammatical skills for writing business letters, and one or two who are mechanically inclined.

Delegating will be less stressful for all concerned if you use tactics that help ensure a successful outcome. This checklist, which will work for someone delegating to a single person or a committee, will lower the risk of mishaps:

- **Know exactly what you want.** Clearly define any specifics you need for a project. For example, if you want a committee to review applications and recommend hires for two field medic positions, outline what's on your mind.

    Tell your committee how many people you want them to interview, what you're looking for in those employees, and any special work experience you'd like to see on a résumé.

- **Match people to the project.** Don't assign casually. Review the training and experience of each delegate. Make sure the person seems right for the work. Plus, his or her schedule should allow enough time to tackle

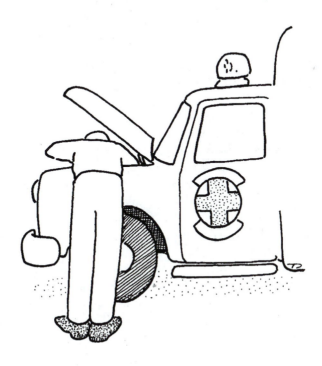

the new assignments. If you're not sure whether someone is willing to take on a new or different job, ask him or her. Enthusiasm for the work should be a factor.

- **Ask for input up front.** Sit down with your delegates and solicit ideas for making something work. Or, ask for suggestions on how to curtail any snags. For example, let's say you have appointed a team to review new equipment purchases. A paramedic might want to voice the pros and cons of a certain brand of rescue harness. Perhaps he or she has worked for another division where the harnesses were used. Encourage active input from this individual.

- **Establish a monitoring system.** You and those you have enlisted should have meetings that serve as checkpoints along the way. If you have three people selecting topics that need to be covered at next month's training sessions, you might review their list on three consecutive Thursday afternoons.

- **Delegate in advance.** As soon as you realize something needs to be done, start planning your delegation process. If individuals or committees have sufficient time to meet a deadline, they'll be more likely to perform the job well. Ample time ensures that they will have more flexibility in their approach, too.

- **Know what *not* to delegate.** Don't delegate tasks that can be performed only at your level of expertise or above. Be aware of what you're expected to perform personally. Example: If your department needs to make a public statement about a controversial incident in your community, don't send an employee to meet the press. Do it yourself.

Respect emotional needs

"I've found myself giving out the same old boring tasks to the same people," explains Harry, a paramedic supervisor who also works as a flight nurse. "It can be tempting to choose the same person over and over because he'll do the job or she'll come through in a pinch. But this is really abusing the privilege of leadership. Finding balance for everyone is the best way to go. And this is greatly achieved through diversifying what everyone does as much as possible."

No one likes to repeat the same old chores without relief. When you delegate, remember to hand out *enjoyable* tasks whenever possible. For example, helping to plan for EMS participation in a local parade or assisting a school with a fair would be fun for some employees. When you pay attention to employees' emotional needs as you delegate, you are helping them to conserve mental energy. Don't repeatedly assign to the same person work that no one else would pick. Spread the aggravation around. It helps to prevent job burnout.

In order to help workers succeed, emphasize hope of success when you delegate. By telling an individual, "I know you'll do a good job," you are setting a positive tone for achievement. However, be sure to set realistic goals for employees. If you assign tasks with unclear outcomes or oversized expectations—like asking a purchasing committee to spend $10,000 for equipment that should run closer to $15,000—you're only setting the stage for frustration.

Reminder

Employees will better support projects they have helped design. By listening to ideas from your personnel, and incorporating as many of those ideas as possible into a project, you are demonstrating your belief in them. Also, remember to find out where each employee wants to go personally. Assign tasks that groom each person for the next rung of the ladder.

If you're good at helping others advance by delegating wisely, should you worry that you will delegate yourself out of a job? After all, what is your job if you give most of your tasks away? Although it can seem scary to empower others, remember that your boss will be impressed if you can bring out the best in others. Top management will always create a position for you if you can do this.

"There are many benefits to good delegating," says Battalion Chief Harold Cohen, who commands the Baltimore County Fire Department in Maryland. "We have over 2,000 employees, and I often give out major assignments. Good delegating helps you evaluate the potential of your personnel."

Cohen believes in the self-directed team approach for delegating large projects. "We appoint teams to study software packages for fire and EMS training, teams to study state laws and the impact they have on our profession, and teams to evaluate medical techniques and equipment," he explains.

He is a firm advocate of the bottom-up versus top-down management style. This means that men and women from the newest ranks are listened to and respected for their ideas. For example, Cohen often places EMTs on committees that have medical experts serving as advisers to the committee. But the EMTs are trusted to solicit information, formulate opinions based on all findings, and advise top management accordingly.

"Certain attitudes work best in handing out assignments to self-directed teams," Cohen asserts. "I tell them to mentally erase the roadblocks in outlining projects. I ask them to be very creative, so they can help move the department forward."

He continues, "It helps to delegate with as few rules as possible. Also, I let my personnel know they'll suffer no negative feedback, if their recommendations differ from my thinking."

"Delegation works best when you let go of preconceived ideas and have positive expectations," he emphasizes. "Sometimes, of course, upper management may have to make changes in the budget a team has outlined. At times, it is necessary to say no to certain ideas. But if progress is to be made in developing your department, you've got to be clear that new ideas are welcome. I tell my men and women that we don't want to continue the weaknesses of the past."

The payoffs are worth it

The long-term effects of good delegating are many. When your personnel learn to carry out new responsibilities on a consistent basis, projects will flow. Besides, any bogged-down projects, or those overlapping in a jam, make you look ineffective as a manager. To avoid this, you can't just put on a "campaign" now and then. You've got to *delegate often to keep the wheels turning.*

Remember that good delegating is one way to affect the financial bottom line. By delegating more and more, you will learn to plan projects of greater value for your division.

As a battalion chief, or a lieutenant in charge of just four people, remember that your worth to your organization lies in maximizing *yourself* as a precious resource, too. Remember that by trying to do everything yourself—without delegating enough—you only wear yourself down.

Moving from underdelegating to adequate delegating takes years for most managers in any type of business. But when you become skilled at planning what to delegate and how, you can even delegate the planning.

As you delegate, it is important to know where to draw the line, however. Never delegate problems that have to do with company morale or serious emotional upsets in the ranks. If you are the top person on the totem pole, let employees know that very stressful situations will be handled by you personally.

If you delegate enough, you'll get a sense of what works and what doesn't. Everybody's strengths and weaknesses will become more apparent. For example, some people will never get the hang of writing a business letter. Conversely, some employees will surprise you with their public speaking skills. But as you entrust others with new projects, they will discover skills they didn't know they had. This enhances each individual's self-confidence.

Job burnout can come from having too few goals—or too many. An employee will feel out of control either way. Delegation should keep *the present workload balanced* and provide stimulating new work.

As a leader, you will earn the respect of others if you help them to learn more and to *become more.* Effective delegation will pave the way for this growth process. Letting go of control does have some risks. But in the long run, the paybacks should far outweigh them.

REVIEW ACTIVITIES

1. Name three ways a leader can empower those he or she supervises. How can empowering others actually reduce a leader's stress in the long run?

2. Why must today's supervisors and managers refute the "tough guy tactics" a leader might have utilized in the past? Why is it important to maintain an attitude of coaching others to succeed?

3. Why are employees one of a company's most valuable assets?

4. As a leader in emergency response, how can you learn to ask questions in a more empowering way when a situation seems difficult to resolve?

5. If you delegated an important assignment to your employees, what is one way you could set up a monitoring system to ensure the project's success?

6. Why is continual delegation more important than putting on a "campaign" now and then?

7. Name five ways a new leader could create a personal plan to sharpen his or her leadership skills.

CLASS PROJECTS

1. Discuss the traits that describe a "superior" leader versus an "average" leader. Are most of these traits related to formal education, one's innate personality, or acquired "people skills"?

2. Discuss personal weaknesses that can alter one's chances for success. How might an individual plan a self-improvement program if he or she is failing to acquire promotions?

CHAPTER SIX

RELATIONSHIPS

"*I was on top of the world," says Julie, a second-generation EMT who works out of a hospital-based EMS station. "My fiancé had just popped the question, and I'd been having the greatest week of my life. I guess I appeared kind of silly because I was smiling so much. Well, I was in the ER with a young boy who'd broken his leg. I was telling some of the nurses about my upcoming June wedding as they attended to our patient."*

She continues, "The ER doctor on duty, who is always stern, apparently didn't like hearing upbeat talk in such a serious setting. After we had the patient taken care of, he looked me straight in the eye and said, 'Young lady, you need to monitor your emotions here in my ER. I want to see you in my office.'"

Julie continues, "I was totally taken aback. I felt nervous as I followed him through the hall to a side room. When I saw what was on his desk, I nearly fainted. This doctor had a huge present wrapped up for me. He told me, 'The staff pitched in on this, but I picked it out. Good luck on your marriage, Julie.' He was the last person on earth I expected this from."

Finding friendships and supportive people is one of the greatest feelings in the world. It is especially nice to have validation from other professionals. Good relationships help us feel that others are interested in our well-being and success. Like Julie, sometimes we are surprised by how positively others feel about us.

Lowering stress levels in all areas of life can be accomplished more effectively when you learn how to participate in relationships. Although you cannot control other people, you can learn how to manage yourself *in relation to others*. Knowing how to interact well with doctors, coworkers, friends, your spouse or significant other, your parents, and your children is imperative for feeling more in control.

Naturally, you want to communicate in ways that enhance each relationship in the long run. For example, you want to have good communication with an ER doctor you see only six times a year. You don't want to work smoothly together on a single occasion—only to find yourselves clashing over an issue the next time you bring a patient to the hospital.

Once you have gained a fair amount of insight into what makes relationships work well, you will intuitively start acting out different behaviors. You may learn to voice a boundary more clearly, or you might begin to state your needs more assertively. By noticing what works and what doesn't in your dealings with each individual, you will gradually learn to act in ways that bring harmony to each relationship. You will also learn how much closeness and how much distance to have with each person in your life.

Although you absolutely cannot control other people—unless you use some type of coercion—you can work with them to find common ground and ward off tension between you. The bottom line is that you want to establish mutual trust. Also, you want to deal with others effectively and still feel good about yourself. You can do this by learning to voice your needs in appropriate ways, perceive the needs of others, set limits with each individual, and interact in ways that help both of you feel okay with the relationship.

Of course, it is hard to set limits with your supervisor or a doctor in charge at the ER, but when other professionals feel they can trust you, it is easier to voice your limits. You gain trust *by being your best self under pressure.* When you learn to bring stability and strength to your EMS team and to your friends and family, they will learn that they can count on you to participate fairly in relationships.

Many of your relationships will be close, even intimate. Others will be friendly, but professional, in tone. Each relationship in your life will be somewhat different from all of the others. With your children, for example, you will have a different chemistry with each child individually. That's because every person in your life brings to your relationship a different set of needs, or a different personal agenda. Each relationship requires a different script to be acted out between the two of you.

However you relate to each individual in your life, you are going to feel happier and more in control with each person *if your core values and beliefs always remain the same.* You don't want to change who you are for every relationship script you must act out in life.

This doesn't mean that your relationship with your parent or child will be the same as with your EMS partner. When you express yourself, you want to feel congruency, or total harmony and inner integrity, about your feelings and actions. You can attain this congruency by speaking and acting out those basic values that you deem important. You want to send identical messages to everyone concerning your integrity and beliefs. Your basic message should say: "I'm giving you respect, and I want respect in return." *Without mutual respect, there is no true relationship going on.*

If you do find yourself in situations where the other person is not respecting you, you need to think about your options. For instance, having a doctor speak rudely to you on several occasions is *not* acceptable. It's your prerogative to meet with those who supervise this doctor at a particular hospital or health-care facility. You can say to this governing body or committee: "There is a problem with one of your doctors. This person is acting out tension and failing to give our staff respect. This is affecting our mutual ability to help our patients. This doctor's attitude is upsetting to me, and it is uncalled for."

Doctors and nurses in the ER are very tired at times, of course, so it is important to give them a break whenever possible. Most of us can get very upset, even hateful, under lots of pressure. This does not mean you should accept cruel or rude behavior as the norm from anyone—even doctors. Doctors are not gods. As an EMT or paramedic, you don't have the same training as a doctor, but you do have areas of expertise that he or she does not have. You have paid your dues in your profession. Your way of presenting yourself should be: "I respect you and your skills, but I need to be respected, also."

EVALUATE YOURSELF FIRST

Before you think about how others treat you in relationships, it is best to take a closer look at how you present yourself. It's true that we teach others how to treat us. But before we can do that, we need to examine how we come across in social and professional situations. After all, if you come across as uncooperative, or as someone with a lack of regard for others, you undoubtedly will be treated the same by some individuals in your life.

But when you change your attitudes and actions in relationships, you will probably find that others start behaving differently toward you. Hopefully, this change on their part will be for the better. There will always be those personality types who are very undiplomatic, of course. There are unkind people in the world who thrive on provoking others. But when you change your behavior for the better and set personal boundaries, you will find it easier to *skirt around difficult people and maintain your balance.*

Reminder

Your goal is not to spend precious time reacting to others. Your goal is to learn how to *respond* appropriately to them. Reacting to someone is very draining and time-consuming. Reacting makes you feel out of control and at the mercy of the other party. Responding in ways that are self-empowering will put energy back into your own life.

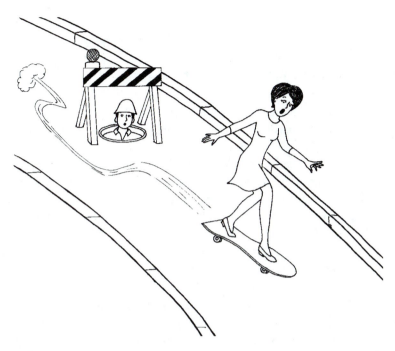

When you become emotionally healthier and better at creating good relationships, you will find yourself attracting emotionally healthier friends and business associates into your life. The old adage that says, "Birds of a feather flock together," is still very true. The reason you want positive, upbeat "birds" in your circle is that you will have stronger, truer allies when things aren't going well for you. Good friends will support you in dozens of ways. For example, if someone at work tries to undermine your efforts, you need allies who will speak up for you. Truly good friends will try to protect you *without hurting or demeaning others.*

Here are some suggestions for acting in more productive and supportive ways to those in your circle of influence:

- **Make sure that you help others feel competent.** No one can feel good in your presence if you continually point out what they lack. Emphasize positive qualities when relating to those around you. It doesn't matter if this person is your cleaning lady or your dental hygienist. If you must point out mistakes or flaws in another's performance at work or at home, do it only after "sandwiching" your criticism between two healthy layers of praise.

    For example, you could tell a coworker: "I always feel our team is on top of things in almost any situation. You do a terrific job. But there is one small thing I need to point out to you. It's just a suggestion. Before you share information with a patient's family, I think you should make sure that the patient is not overhearing some of the things you say." Then tell your coworker the specifics of what he or she did wrong. Follow this up by saying, "You're always trying hard to do a good job, and I feel you need to know this."

- **Practice being agreeable.** Sometimes it is tempting to make a lot of negative comments. But if you act, think, and talk in a more agreeable way, you are going to find more grounding in all of your relationships. This is partly due to the fact that *you will feel more in control of yourself* when you're in a more positive mode.

    Besides, people in your life will subconsciously "rate" their relationship with you according to how you make them feel when they are in your presence. Do you drag other people down? Do you drone on about your personal problems? Then you are also making your listener participate in this misery. All of us share problems, but if you talk too negatively, your listener will consciously or subconsciously build wider boundaries between you. This will make it hard for you to have a close relationship with this person.

- **Ask other people what they need from you.** Of course, this must be done wisely. You wouldn't ask someone what he or she needs if this individual has a reputation of taking advantage of others. You wouldn't unless you enjoy having dependent people in your life. But in most of your relationships, it will be safe to offer small amounts of assistance or cooperation without bending yourself out of shape.

    For example, if you spend time with a friend, remember to ask: "Where would you like to go this afternoon?" or "Do you need to borrow any of my books on creating Web pages for the Internet?" It's easy to forget that other people have agendas, too. Most of us can't wait to tell others our problems, our needs, our peeves. But a good relationship must be a two-way street *where the give and take between both parties feels balanced.*

If you're a supervisor, it is good to occasionally ask your employees: "How can I help you succeed? Do you need something from me?"

"INTIMATE RELATIONSHIP" SAVVY

Managing personal stress levels will be easier, also, if you understand more about how to create good intimate relationships. Nothing is quite so unnerving as a love relationship that is strained.

For example, Shelley, a flight nurse–paramedic who works one full-time job and one part-time job, says, "My husband and I don't have time to work on our marriage. We are both so stressed out that we have nothing left to give when we get home. We argue a lot, and this really scares me. After an argument, sometimes we're cold toward each other for days. We both want a good marriage, but we're each in a position where we have to give a lot to our careers. How can we hold it all together, when we're this exhausted?"

Emergency responders can learn to have good marriages and good relationships. This will mean acquiring skills for better communication. In fact, the more stressful your job, the better your communication skills should be within your marriage. After all, the quality of your relationship with someone is really *the quality of your conversation* with that person—whether spouse, child, or coworker. Conversation is always both spoken and unspoken.

In Shelley's case, for example, frequent arguing is, of course, not good communication. In fact, married couples can argue because they fear losing touch with each other. Arguing can be a subconscious, but desperate, way of saying, "We need to stay connected." Acting cold toward a spouse for days after an argument sends all kinds of messages, too. For example, pulling back inside your own space by becoming silent and distant tells your partner, "I don't like you very much right now."

Figuring out how to navigate smoothly within a relationship is something that has puzzled intimate partners down through the ages. Of course, the common question we've all heard that most men have is *What do women want?* The common question women have about intimate relationships is *Why won't men open up and talk?*

Most emergency responders do want intimacy with a spouse or significant other. But attaining closeness with a partner can be complicated, if not totally elusive. Deep down, most of us know that a good relationship helps to cushion the stress of life. But the stress levels experienced by individuals in public safety jobs or the health-care field can make it hard to be emotionally available for a mate at times. How can you give of yourself emotionally to another when your resources have been so depleted?

After a killer shift, all you probably want to do is get out of your work clothes and collapse. You want quiet time by yourself to decompress. Having a mate or a child who requires attention can make you think: "Don't make any demands! I just want to be left alone!" But when you learn to discuss your feelings more openly, you can ease the transition from work to home.

You might tell your family, "Come close and let me hold all of you for a minute. Then please, give me 45 minutes by myself. I need this time, or I'm going to be irritable and cranky. We'll talk after I calm down a bit."

When you can verbalize a boundary with your family this way, you're saying, "I want to touch base, and after I've had my quiet time, we will reconnect." Act positive about what you require. Your family will learn to adjust if you tell them, "I can give more, if I get settled down. Thanks for helping me do this." It *is* important to reconnect physically with each member, even if you can spend only five minutes of uninterrupted time with each child and fifteen minutes of one-on-one time with your spouse. Focus on each individual. Make the connection a true moment of quality time. If you don't feel like talking, say to each family member, "Tell me about your day. I'm listening."

Remember that *others bond with you when you actively listen to them.* They do not necessarily bond when you do all the talking. Bonding takes place when someone feels you are on the receiving end, absorbing their thoughts and feelings. So if you are exhausted, you can still help your mate or your child feel that time spent with you is quality time. Focus on the other person, even for a short time.

Phillip, a firefighter in his mid-thirties shares this story about his family: "My kids used to come running outside to meet my car when I'd get home. Well, I'd hit the kitchen and my wife would be in a talkative mood. She'd start in with this chattering about the kids, her day, the problems, the bills. I hate to say this, but I wanted to dive back in the car and flee! I love my wife, but talking a lot is the last thing I can stand when I'm tired. Finally, I had to tell her, 'Honey, I can't bear to have to listen this much when I'm wiped out. I know you need to talk. But please don't talk a lot when I first hit the door.' "

He continues, "Of course, it hurt her feelings. There's no easy way to tell anyone to cool it on the talking bit. But after she got over her mad spell, I just reiterated what I'd said before. I told her, 'I'm not trying to hurt our relationship. But you've got to respect my limits here when I first get home. I need the house to be quiet, until I can pull myself together.' She finally understood. To show my appreciation, I always hug her for a long time after I get calmed down. I might not want to talk, but I do embrace her for a good long time.

"I think a lot of relationships go down the tubes because men, especially, will not tell their wives what the real problems are. And I'm sure there are women who don't spell out what they need. But for me, when I could just tell my wife the truth about the situation, I knew I was on the right track to helping our relationship. Speaking for myself, I think that finding the words to express what I need from my wife—and praying she won't get mad at me—is the hardest part of my relationship with her."

Learning to have a good relationship with most of the people in your life will require that you can ask for what you need. Like Phillip, most of us know that they may get angry with us. After all, we're asking them to change their behavior. This is no small thing. Asking that a need be met can also be a form of setting a boundary. We have to tell the other person, "What you're doing isn't going to work anymore. I can't allow this or that to continue without speaking up."

Choosing the words to voice a need is hard for most of us. Unless we grow up in a family where good communication is modeled, it can be hard to speak well in a tense situation. It is almost impossible to model behavior you've never seen. If your family of origin did not have good communication skills, you will probably find it difficult to acquire them.

Let's say that your parents did not communicate well. If you have acquired good communication skills, it's probably because you somehow learned to model those skills from other people in your sphere of influence. Perhaps you learned from friends, teachers, or coworkers.

However, if you feel you are lacking in good relationship know-how, you can still learn productive interaction by working on one or two skills at a time. After you get a handle on managing one or two improvements, you can find more ways to communicate effectively and work on your relationships. Eventually, you will get the knack of how to interact well in almost all social and professional circles.

Whereas some relationships begin and end in one afternoon, such as getting to know a patient, most relationships are ongoing. You always have an opportunity to keep improving them. The chemistry between yourself and a child, a mate, or a coworker can become less strained, even harmonious. Although you can't really change or fix others, you can learn to interact in ways that help you feel better about yourself. One excellent way to judge whether you are playing fair in a relationship is to pretend that you are being videotaped. If others watched the tape, would they think you were acting wisely? Would they perceive that you were trying hard not to invade or injure the boundaries of the other party?

If your marriage is in trouble, there are still lots of opportunities for turning things around. Of course, your mate has to be willing to work with you. Remember Chad in Chapter 2? He and his wife sought support from a counselor. They then wrote a contract for improving their marriage. They agreed to implement one new relationship skill per week. They decided to work on listening to each other the first week, work on setting boundaries the second week, and progress to polishing other skills thereafter.

All of your relationships can be improved by this method. Much of the change is up to you. When you demonstrate good communication skills, you are teaching others how you want to be treated. For instance, are you helping other people to feel valued? Are you listening well? Do you let your spouse and children know that you want to be there for them, even if you can't do a perfect job of looking after their needs?

MARRIAGE TIPS THAT WORK

Couples under stress can have a good relationship by actively working on changes that benefit both partners. According to Willard F. Harley Jr., Ph.D., author of *Give and Take: The Secret to Marital Compatibility* (Revell, 1996), the most productive way to accomplish this is for couples to incorporate what he calls a "policy of joint agreement" into their marriage.

"The policy states that you should never do anything without an enthusiastic agreement between you and your spouse," Dr. Harley explains. This means that every time you do something both of you must enthusiastically agree or you don't do it. He continues, "For example, when planning a vacation, both of you must negotiate where you're going and how you'll be spending your time until you're both enthusiastic about the plan."

Dr. Harley contends that this policy is easy to implement in marriages that are already doing great. But couples who are struggling see this policy as not only difficult, but crazy. This is because they are not in the habit of taking each other's feelings into account when they make decisions. According to Dr. Harley, that's precisely why they are not doing well.

Dr. Harley has found that if these struggling couples force themselves to use the policy of joint agreement, it becomes easier and easier to implement. The easier it becomes, the better the marriage gets.

However, he cautions, many couples find the policy of joint agreement difficult to follow during the first week. "To help couples understand how the policy works, I ask them to practice in areas that are not very important to them, such as grocery shopping," he points out. "For example, the couple can walk up and down the aisles of the grocery store—selecting only items for the cart that they both can enthusiastically agree to purchase. If one spouse wants an item and the other is not enthusiastic about it, they must negotiate with each other *until the reluctant spouse becomes enthusiastic* or the item is left on the shelf.

"At first, a couple may find that there aren't too many items in the cart following a tour of the store," he continues. "But after they improve their negotiating skills, they find that they can fill the cart."

He summarizes: "By using these same negotiating skills that lead to an enthusiastic agreement, couples can learn to resolve some of their most difficult conflicts."

> *Tammy, mother of two, who is a nurse at a large community hospital, points out why* not *having a policy of joint agreement has hurt her marriage. "My husband has gotten our two sons involved in all kinds of sports," she explains. "He doesn't consult with me on their activities at all. If they have a game, he gets angry if I can't make arrangements to take them. I believe my husband is living too much through our children, instead of making friends of his own. He gets a lot out of these games, but the children and I are worn out. He refuses to discuss the situation."*

> *Jake, a police officer who is now in a second marriage, says that he and his first wife were always pulling in opposite directions on problems. They couldn't get the hang of working on solutions they both could support. "My first marriage failed because we didn't have the patience or skills to figure out how both of us could be happy," he confesses. "In my present marriage, things are different. My wife, Janna, came into this marriage saying, 'We have to talk about our problems and work out good solutions.'"*

He continues, *"I'll give you an example of what it takes for us to find a good plan. Janna's mother was in the hospital last year. At this same time, I wanted to go on a four-day fishing trip with two of my friends. Let me tell you, no woman wants to hear that you'll be having fun while her mother is sick. Well, I needed the vacation badly. I'd had a rough stretch of working two homicides and a drive-by shooting."*

Jake and Janna were able to come up with a workable plan, so that each felt okay about it. "I stopped by the hospital to tell my mother-in-law why I needed a break," Jake explains. "I made it clear to her that I would come home from my trip if she had any complications. Also, I asked her to spend two weeks at our house after she was released from the hospital. My children and I shared the duties of taking care of her, along with my wife and my stepdaughter. I was mentally rested after my fishing trip, so everything worked out well for all of us.

"My wife and I have worked out other similar problems with extended family in the past. We also have tricky problems with both of our ex-spouses which arise. Janna and I have become quite good at figuring out how to meet our mutual needs and take care of others in the process. Stepfamilies, especially, have to work diligently at this."

Because marriage today involves more complex role requirements than it might have 30 or 40 years ago, couples need to become very good at *creating solutions*. It helps to address problems from several standpoints, too. If one solution doesn't work, there's no reason why you cannot try another.

Christy, a wife and mother of two-year-old twins, was having a rough time managing a full-time job with two toddlers. She was exhausted working 53 hours a week as a paramedic in a busy section of town. "My husband, Doug, made it clear he did not want me to quit, because our budget was very tight," Christy explains. "Both of our cars needed work, and we needed to buy a bigger house. Doug and I decided we'd figure out creative ways to get my stress and our money problems under control."

She explains: "My boss was inflexible about my working part-time, so I asked Doug to approach his boss about a change in his work schedule. Doug works at a retail store. His boss agreed to let him off on Tuesdays and Thursdays, if he'd work weekends. I'm off on Tuesdays and Thursdays, so Doug watches the children while I catch up on sleep. I asked my mother to help out a few hours on Saturday, and Doug's sister helps out on Sundays. It gives me the breathing room I need to manage the children and a stressful job. We'll do this for a while, until I can get transferred to a quieter substation across town. The twins will be older then, and they should be easier to manage."

Christy says their money problems eased somewhat when Doug asked his boss to let him drive a used company car. "It really helped when his boss agreed to this," Christy continues. "We sold one of our cars to get rid of the monthly payment of two hundred dollars. With the extra money, we were able to finance a much bigger house. We improved our lives because we were willing to ask for help from our relatives and Doug's boss. You've got to create what you want in your mind, and then make it happen."

Couples who avidly seek better solutions to their problems are going to create better lives for their children as well. Children benefit when they see you dealing with problems in a very innovative and positive way. If they see you working out good solutions, they will grow up believing they can, too.

Dr. Edward Mahoney, director of graduate counseling programs at Notre Dame College in Manchester, New Hampshire, points out that good communication skills do not come naturally for most couples. "We must consciously learn how to interact and solve problems," he states. "Couples who can do this feel more secure. Those who can't often feel isolated in their marriages."

Here are further tips for making your marriage work:

- **Make a true pact that you want a good marriage.** If you want to learn how to solve problems in your marriage, you have to recognize this *as a skill that takes practice.* But you can't practice all by yourself. Actively enlist your spouse's help. Ask him or her, "Would you agree that we need to work at communicating?" Don't just get a nod of agreement, though. A true pact involves saying "Are you giving me a solemn commitment here?"

- **Set some rules together.** A good place to start is by saying, "We'll try to use pleasant voice tones," or "We'll try not to interrupt each other." Practice only one or two rules at a time to keep yourself on track.

- **Provide a clue word.** Agree upon a word or a phrase to let your partner know that you need to talk over an issue. You could say, "Let's have a powwow," or "Let's hit the sofa for a chat."

  Don't overuse your signal for needing a private conference, however. Don't have a long talk over which table lamps to buy, unless you have loads of free time. Save your talks for important problems.

- **Learn what a need is.** A need, which is a desire that often has been with you since childhood, can be connected to almost any problem you have. Identifying your needs will take careful thought and self-awareness. It's okay to want a need acknowledged, even if it seems a little selfish to someone else.

  For instance, if you need to have a neat house, it is important to tell your partner, "We need to find ways to store things and keep the house looking better. I need you to take this seriously. Could we devise a better plan that will work for both of us?"

Be proactive

It is important to help your mate succeed at pleasing you. Boldly asserting yourself might be a real stretch for you. But if you are pleasant and upbeat about it, what do you have to lose? For instance, if you expect gifts on holidays, circle these dates on the calendar and speak up a few days ahead of time. Tell your spouse, "I need to feel special, and I'm making it easy for you to remember that." If your budget is tight, he or she can always cook dinner at home and take you out for a nice dessert. A gift can be inexpensive. But make it clear that it is the attention you crave.

> *Another proactive tip is this: When you interact with your spouse or significant other, use your "pause" button frequently. It takes willpower to keep quiet, but sometimes keeping quiet is the very thing to do to attain control. Practice waiting before you jump in with comments. Don't interject your thoughts and feelings into the context of what he or she has stated. Pause, think, and then offer an opinion. This way, your spouse won't feel so threatened by your opinions or input.*

KEEPING RELATIONSHIPS HEALTHY

There is almost an infinite number of skills any of us could learn in managing relationships. But there are some basic guidelines for how to maintain relationships. When you think about your relationship with a friend, marriage partner, or coworker, remember these suggestions for how to participate in relationships:

- **Never use relationships to give yourself self-esteem.** Needing too much approval from others will have you acting inappropriately for yourself. For example, you might find yourself volunteering to do things you don't want to do because you need someone's validation. Confusion and frustration will cloud any relationship if you expect the wrong things from it.

  As much as you care for your family members and friends, you must demonstrate self-worth by acting confidently about what you value. You should feel good about yourself by being exactly who you want to be without worrying too much if others will put their stamp of approval on you.

- **Good relationships don't require that we feel other people's emotions for them.** If others overwhelm you with their problems, realize that offering a listening ear and giving emotional support won't drain you. But doing someone else's "emotional work" for them will. If you do want to help someone, offer to do something very specific for an individual. You might offer someone a ride home, or you might offer to help someone find an apartment. But just "feeling" another's burdens won't help anything.

- **A relationship is not healthy if you can't give it a bottom line on how you'll participate.** For example, you can decide that you'll go out to dinner once a month with a friend. However, don't let your friend unload emotionally for hours on the phone with you. If your inner voice tells you, "I am not getting enough respect in this relationship," you should heed what you're hearing. Find a way to voice your bottom line on how much you can give or do.

- **Act for yourself in a relationship, not to control the other party.** For example, if you need to share information with your mate or significant other, try to express yourself in a way that feels right to you—not to force the other person to cooperate.

    For instance, if your in-laws want you and your spouse to visit every single weekend, you might not feel comfortable with this schedule. You can always tell your spouse, "I want you to visit your parents every Saturday if you like. That's fine. But my free time is so limited I don't feel I can go every weekend."

SETTING BOUNDARIES

Learning to get along well with others will require you to learn skills for setting clearly defined boundaries. You must be able to tell another person what you can give or do.

Also, you need to listen to your inner voice about each person's behavior. We all have instincts about other people, and we can get into real trouble when we ignore what our inner voice tells us about them. Decide very carefully about the degree of closeness you want with someone.

In order to navigate successfully within any relationship, you must be able to (verbally and assertively) set boundaries with the other party. Otherwise, the boundary lines will become blurred. If your skills in this area have never been up to par, this takes lots of practice. It is quite difficult to set boundaries if you did not hear your parents or family members "draw a line in the sand" for others in a healthy and nonoffensive way.

The following suggestions can get you on the right track:

- **First define the limit that feels reasonable for you.** If you're working full time and taking classes at night, you might not feel you can visit your child's classroom every week. Maybe his or her teacher wants your help in grading papers and tutoring some of the children in reading skills.

You feel some guilt because you know your child enjoys your visits, but every week is too much for your schedule. However, you need to ask yourself what would feel right. Could you help out every third or fourth week for two or three hours? Or, could you spend one full day in the classroom once each month?

- **Start by setting small boundaries.** Learn to verbalize something as simple as this: "I need to get off the phone. I've got so much I need to do." Keep working at voicing your limits to others. If possible, move slowly and give the other party time to adjust to your limits. As you perfect your boundary-setting skills, you will learn how firm your boundaries need to be. Only by practicing how to set limits can you be firm with patients, coworkers, or friends *without sounding offensive;* you are training yourself to be assertive rather than aggressive.

- **Expect every boundary you set to be tested.** People often will try to get you to remove the limit you have set by certain things they say or do. When you draw a line by setting a limit, the other person may give back this message: "I've heard your boundary, but I don't like it. I liked the old way better."

Expect to have countermoves from each person who will verbally or nonverbally say, "Change back to the way you were. I don't like your boundary. It doesn't make life comfortable for me."

- **Practice what you will say, so you won't be caught off guard.** For example, your best friend may complain if you don't visit every week. You might practice a response such as: "I'd love to come over, but there are certain classes I really need to take right now. I hope you understand that I miss our time together, but for now, I have to make this sacrifice. Please bear with me on this situation."

Don't expect anyone to love you for making necessary changes. People want you to stay the same *so they can stay the same.* They have enjoyed the predictability you provided up to this point. When you put a limit on something, this means that your coworker, spouse, or friend will have to find a substitute, or alternative, for what you have been providing. But if a change is necessary to protect your deepest interests and values, stick with it.

Friendships require respect

"I've been an EMS supervisor since the early '70s," says Frank, a firefighter who has taught at several community colleges. "One of the biggest problems I've

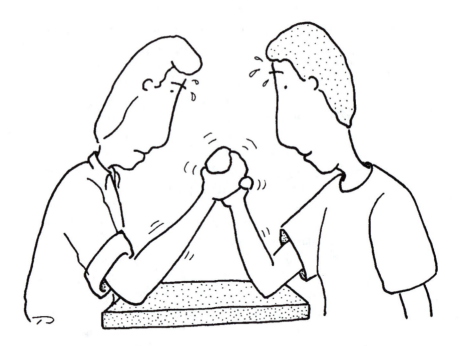

found in this line of work is that some paramedics like to compete in the wrong areas. In the work setting, they want to "one-up" everybody on this call or that call. They want to review somebody's call sheet and say, 'I could have done it faster. I would have done it differently.' Now, it doesn't take a genius to figure out that this is not the way to create a good feeling between two fellow workers."

Frank continues, "Men, especially, have been taught to compete from the time they were old enough to crawl. They don't have the bonding and friendship skills that women do. Some do, but most don't. That's why men get out on a limb. When they need to share pain or some marital problem, they don't have a close friend to go to. Very few men routinely confide in another male friend about personal problems. And they probably don't have an in-depth chat like women have. Men are scared to death that something they say can be used against them."

It is true that men can feel very isolated when problems occur because most do refrain from sharing sensitive issues with other men. To complicate matters, men often fear sharing problems openly with their wives or girlfriends. This can be because they don't want to appear vulnerable, or they may fear that *their problems will not be kept confidential.* After all, it is common knowledge that women bond by sharing secrets about their private lives. So this leaves men in a double bind. They don't feel comfortable sharing problems with a man or a woman!

It is very important for women to understand that men need confidantes. Men also need to help women understand that private matters are private. When women learn how much men need to be listened to and understood, men will feel much safer in opening up to them about problems. Men can learn to tell a wife, sister, or mother: "I need to share some of my thoughts with you. I can't do that unless you promise me that you will not talk about this with other people."

When women fully understand how sensitive men really are about personal issues, they can become better friends to their husbands, sons, brothers, and coworkers. Women can help relieve a lot of stress by remembering some of the basic needs of men and boys.

The following tips can give a man insight into *how to share with a woman what she needs to know* about intimate conversations with a male. These suggestions can also help women get a clearer vision of what males need from them. If you are chosen as a confidante to a male, remember to follow these guidelines:

- **Actively listen to him.** Men feel closer to those who refrain from talking too much and who attentively absorb what they have to say. It can be tempting to jump in with advice, criticism, or needs of your own, but hold off and let him talk. A man's stress compounds when he has no verbal outlet for his emotions.

    Whereas women usually engage in "girl talk" several times a week with women friends, studies show that only one in ten men has a really close friend. Men need the luxury of being heard. Males usually associate in groups. When a man has more than one friend, each friend knows only a little about him. Therefore, if a man chooses you— whether you are male or female—as his continual sounding board, there's a good chance that *you're the only person who really listens to him at all.*

- **Show respect for what he values.** This is the shortest route to building a solid emotional bond with a male, whether he's your husband, brother, or son. For example, when you support your husband's love of auto racing or growing prize tomatoes, you're validating him as a person.

    Your husband or son will become extremely frustrated if he can't share his true self with his family. It is hard for males to feel connected to those who don't show respect for their special likes and dislikes. As trite as it sounds, boys and men want others in their families to know small things such as their food preferences. Whereas females enjoy being a little mysterious at times, males deeply crave *to be understood* by those close to them.

- **See him as a man, not a hero.** Contrary to what young girls learn from *Cinderella* and other fairy tales, men do not want to be viewed as solutions to women's problems. The more problems a wife verbalizes, *the more inadequate and helpless a man feels.*

Men don't want to be cast in a Superman role, because they know they can't live up to it. Naturally, women deserve and need specific help from their husbands and sons. But females should approach a male in the same thoughtful way they would approach a female friend for help—with full consideration for his time and energy levels.

The silent treatment

Adult males who are under stress often distance themselves from their coworkers, wives, and children by constructing a wall of silence. Some men express such distancing behavior by drinking too much or having extramarital affairs. When these men cite stress at home as an excuse for some hurtful act, such as having an affair, they often feel justified in what they have done. This isn't because men are uncaring or insensitive to others. Men can simply reach a point where they believe that their emotional needs *do not matter* to their wives or to their friends.

"Males under stress tend to act in very rigid ways," says Du Bois Williams, Ph.D., who teaches clinical psychology at Xavier University in New Orleans. "They're protecting their egos."

Females act out tension also, but they usually are quicker to seek reconnection with family and friends after distancing. Males tend to stay in an isolated mode longer, because they don't know how to reach out for consolation the way females do.

Due to social conditioning and genetic differences, males tend to be very solution oriented. They want to fix things quickly. When they can't, they may become very frustrated and *angry with themselves.* That's why giving advice to a man can backfire, unless he openly asks for your opinion. A man can lose a sense of feeling in control when advice is lavished on him. To a male under stress, well-meant advice can feel like criticism.

Try these suggestions when a male coworker, your brother, or your husband confides that his stress is escalating:

- **Remind him to look at his options.** Males often believe that they don't have any options. They don't usually reflect on problems in a broader context the way females do. Women usually bounce problems off of lots of people in order to get a feel for possible solutions.

    When a male employee, your father, or your son has a problem, encourage him to think of several ways to approach it. For example, if he is getting drained from overwork, suggest that he might think of three ways to manage his time better.

- **Point out that giant leaps don't work.** Because males like to fix things quickly, it's good to remind your male EMS partner or your son that he should tackle complicated problems slowly. Using small, manageable steps that break a problem down into easy parts works best.

  Quantum leaps seldom work, except in fantasy stories about male heroes. Although these heroes with quick-fix abilities are interesting, they are false role models.

- **Offer to be there for him.** When a problem nags at your teenage son or your father, he'll feel your support if you assure him, "I'll be here if you need me." Make sure he knows he's free to bounce ideas off you, even if you don't have any solutions for his problems.

What do women need?

Men can stay so confused about how to converse with a female who's under pressure that they just give up. A woman, without meaning to, can overwhelm a man when she talks about her difficulties. Although she is just getting things off her mind, a man can think she expects him to fix her problems. If her problems are complex, this can make him feel out of control.

Men who have grown up in a household with at least one sister probably feel more comfortable chatting with females. For one thing, they learn that women enjoy sharing feelings very openly. These men know that women don't necessarily expect anyone to fix their anxieties. They just like to share what's on their mind with someone they trust. Many women will share much more information than the average man cares to hear!

There are several theories about why women talk more than men. One of them is this: From the beginning of time, men learned to talk less because of their role as hunters. Two men chatting in the woods might scare off a deer or other game. Too much verbal interaction could mean a man's family could starve.

On the other hand, women were primarily "gatherers" up until recent decades. They were left alone to harvest herbs and vegetables while the men hunted. As women worked the fields or gathered herbs in the woods, they talked a lot to warn wild animals away. Talking was essentially a matter of life or death for women down through the ages.

Whether or not you agree with this theory, or you have a better one of your own, the fact is that women utter more sounds than men. Because women use language more, they often have an advantage over men during a conversation. If a man can think of one reason he doesn't want to do something, a woman can quickly list a dozen reasons why he should do it! Small wonder a man will keep quiet and "go into his cave" when the heat is on in an argument with a female.

Because of different conversational styles, men can feel very disadvantaged when helping women who are under stress. "I used to feel like a woman just wanted to dump on me and ruin my day," laughs Denver, an ER doctor. "My strategy is to address a problem, solve it, and move on to the next thing. I used to think some of the women I dated were weird because they talked so much about their problems. No wonder I was single for years!"

He continues, "I can laugh about that now. I was an only child, so I didn't understand how females worked through issues. I didn't have any sisters, and my mom is a real quiet lady. When I hit 30, I started reading books on relationships. I've read enough to know that women need to vent their problems. It's just their way of releasing pressure and getting a handle on things."

Denver, who is now a happily married father, is right about most women having a *need* to talk. Sharing a problem with a good listener feels wonderful to a female.

In order to help a female under stress—whether she's your EMS partner, your daughter, or your sister—keep these points in mind:

- **A woman's initial "venting" is an unwinding session.** Whereas men thrive on hearing logic, women thrive on *describing their feelings.* Woman find it comforting to say almost anything they can think of when they're under stress.

    Phrases such as "I'm going nuts" or "My life is miserable" are often just figures of speech for a stressed-out female. She doesn't need fixing or rescuing. She just needs an active listener. If in doubt about how worried she really is, ask her: "How bad is this problem on a scale of one to 10? Are you asking for any specific help, or do you just need to vent?"

- **Women vent *more* when they can't define the true problem.** For example, females can struggle to understand the behavior of those around them. Keeping family members bonded has been of primary concern to females down through the ages. When there are problems involving people, women typically view the problem from more angles than men do. This can cause *women themselves* a lot of frustration.

    Help a woman to define the true problem behind her worries, if this is possible at the time. Or, bear with her if it isn't possible. Lacey, a paramedic from Alabama, shares this story: "I was worried about a single man on our shift who seemed depressed. I wondered if he might be ill or in some kind of personal trouble. The guys on our shift couldn't understand why I was worrying over this man. They looked at me like I was the one with the problem."

- **If she defines very specific problems, suggest a plan of action.** Women sometimes need to be reminded, as do men, that a plan of action will reduce stress. Whereas men immediately think about *how* to fix a problem—if they can find an option or solution—women can forget to be solution oriented at all.

Women experience their problems in such a deeply personal way that they sometimes live inside a problem for days or weeks. They can become enmeshed in the problem as they talk about it and think about it. But they are not necessarily fixated on finding an immediate solution the way most men are. Men want to fix things fast. Women need to process slowly.

Listening to anyone—male or female—about the same old problems over and over can be draining. As a listener, you do have the right to call a halt to being an emotional dumping ground. Gently remind the complainer that implementing a good plan will save energy. Try something such as this: "I'm very clear on your problem, and you certainly have a right to feel badly about this. However, you're not getting anywhere. What kind of action is going to help you? Have you thought about solutions that are really going to help?"

Bailey, a police officer in New England, helped his wife get a plan of action going when her job became overwhelming. "My wife kept telling me how tired she was," says Bailey. "She was working 75 hours each week at a desk job. I ignored her grumbling at first. I'd let it go in one ear and out the other. But when I really listened, I saw that she was being crushed by her work.

"I said to her one night: 'Ask your boss to hire a part-time assistant for you.'" She looked dumbstruck. She said, 'Should I do that?' It was as if she didn't know she could invent a solution. The company she works for isn't stingy or uncaring. What shocked me was the fact she hadn't thought of this on her own. When we have a problem, it can feel a little too good to nurse the problem, instead of pinning down a real solution. Well, my wife asked for an assistant and got a great one."

If your wife or significant other is challenged by your long hours and lack of emotional support, help her to define a way to develop good support. Work with her on creating options that take pressure off her. "I used to agonize a lot because my husband worked such long hours," says Meagan, a young wife who attends college full-time. "I didn't get married to be abandoned. My husband, who works two jobs as a paramedic, has tried to be supportive."

She continues, "He has encouraged me to have friends over, work out at the college gym, and fight my loneliness. I can find ways to deal with the loneliness. But it's easier when he says, 'I know you're lonely, and I'm here to help you deal with it.' When a husband really cares about a wife's problem and helps her work on it, it really takes some of the pain out of it."

Confusion about roles

Since the women's movement began, men have experienced lots of stress within their own families. Their main complaint is that they find it hard to juggle all of the roles they are expected to play. Many women have expanded their roles by choice. But men have been forced to expand theirs. Although these changes are good and necessary, men say it is difficult to adapt.

"It's tough to model a version of a man you've never seen," says Kenneth, 41, father of three who is a physician's assistant. "All I ever saw my father do was go to his factory job and play a little golf occasionally. He didn't have any challenging goals. He didn't have a large network of friends, except for acquaintances at church. And above all, my father did not help my mother around the house."

Kenneth continues, "My wife and I used to argue constantly about my not helping with the kids and the housework. I've had to work hard to be a modern version of a man." Kenneth says that figuring out how to help his wife take care of the kids, the chauffeuring and the household chores after a full day at work was almost impossible. "Heck, it's nearly killed me to get the hang of it," he laughs.

As men struggle to adjust to their complex roles, women are finding it equally hard to adjust. Their roles as working wives with children or working single mothers leave them feeling exhausted and unsupported at times. For women who have ambitions about rising to the top in their companies, they are finding it hard to break through the "glass ceiling" to top management jobs.

It is not easy for anyone to maneuver through all of the adjustments within the changing family or the changing workplace. But by networking with people from all walks of life, you can gather more ideas about how to make your life work. You can "borrow" strategies from different role models in order to plan how you will function within your role as employee, friend, parent, or marriage partner.

"I used to wonder how my supervisor accomplished so much in his personal life," says Allen, an EMT from Indiana. "I was struggling to manage my job, a small apartment, and a girlfriend I saw two nights a week. It was that period of life where I was struggling to get my laundry done, socialize a little, sleep, and make it to work on time. My supervisor had a wife, three children, and did lots of volunteer work, in addition to his hours at our EMS station.

"What I learned by socializing with my boss was that he accomplished a lot by focusing. He didn't talk about work in the car with me, and he didn't think about EMS matters on his family's time. It's helped me see that you have to focus like a laser beam on doing your work well. Then you have to refocus on what else you want to do. Now I'm happily married and expecting a child. I use my boss as a role model. Some of the men and women at work accuse me of trying to gain favors by running around with the boss. Well, he did me a very large favor. He's provided me with a good role model and friend rolled into one. I don't care what the people at work say."

DESTRUCTIVE RELATIONSHIPS

Although some individuals such as Allen do get lucky enough to have a great boss–friend, there will be a time in almost everyone's life when a *destructive* boss, friend, coworker, or mate is in the picture. Whether you are male or female, you may have to make a major change in your life regarding a particular relationship at some point. You may have to ask for a transfer to a different fire or EMS station in order to escape a coworker or boss you can't tolerate. Or, you may find yourself wanting to escape a bad love relationship. You may need to end a relationship with a dating partner or a marriage partner.

Although it probably is best to back away from destructive relationships slowly, this may not always be an option. Sometimes, you have to announce, "I want out." If you are in a situation where you're not getting respect, and it is not likely that you will ever get it, it can be best to end the relationship before it costs you too much emotionally.

Whereas ending a bad relationship at work can be as simple as quietly asking for a transfer, your ending a relationship with a close friend or intimate partner can be difficult. Ending a marriage is something you should consider only after professional counseling. But ending a relationship with a destructive *dating partner* can require professional guidance, too. EMS, police, and fire personnel can get involved in dating situations in which the other person is possessive, even dangerous.

If you answer yes to the following questions, you probably are in a relationship that isn't healthy:

- Do you often have to abandon your routine to respond to the selfish needs of your partner?
- Are you preoccupied with each other's behavior?
- Are you dependent on each other's approval for a sense of self-worth?
- Is there jealousy and possessiveness coming from one or both of you?

For example, some public safety providers and emergency responders report that their husbands and wives are extremely jealous of their professional partners.

Although some jealousy is normal, it is important to be aware of extreme jealousy, which could escalate into an abusive situation.

No one should end an intimate relationship casually. In fact, it is important to take responsibility for trying to improve it, if possible. Try to talk about what a healthier relationship would involve with your spouse or significant other. If physical abuse ever enters the picture, you *should not* try to fix the relationship without the help of a counselor. If your partner is willing to talk openly with you, there may be some hope. However, if your partner goes into denial about the abuse, there is no hope that the relationship will get better.

A healthier relationship with a member of the opposite sex would involve such things as the following:

- **Each partner should desire that the other grow as a person.** Both partners should celebrate each other's successes.
- **Each has a strong sense of "self" that does not come from the other person.** An intimate partnership should mean that you are "bonded" instead of "blended." Both people should maintain a healthy *separate* identity that comes from having personal values, beliefs, and goals that are uplifting and productive.
- **Each has the encouragement of the other to maintain healthy friendships outside of the relationship.** Same-sex friendships help each partner to feel balanced within a close love relationship. This is because boundaries are more softened in a love relationship. Such closeness can throw anyone a little off balance *because of being vulnerable to another person.* Healthy friendships for each partner will provide support and comfort in a way one's intimate partner cannot.

HELPING A SIGNIFICANT OTHER OR COWORKER UNDER STRESS

In every close relationship, each individual will watch the other person endure stressful situations. Our mates or significant others will experience job stress, problems with their families of origin, or financial difficulties. Many spouses or significant others of EMS workers say that they need coping tools for helping their partners when stress intensifies.

Marriages and intimate relationships can become destructive when one partner is caught up in a stressful state. This can take the form of grouchiness, depression, withdrawal, or emotional outbursts. This is not to say that any of us can psychoanalyze or fix someone we care about. We don't have that kind of power. However, it is possible to help an individual under severe stress weigh options, think more clearly, and figure out how to make a plan for positive results.

"Of course you must already have that kind of closeness in place," says Linda Honeycutt, an EMS coordinator for a hospital in the Detroit, Michigan, area. "You can't sit down and have this kind of one-on-one conversation if you haven't been close in the first place."

Honeycutt has been a paramedic for 23 years and an educator since 1980. She has taught classes on EMS stress management that offer information about the basic personality of emergency service providers. "Significant others need to understand that many police, fire, and EMS personnel tend to have a perfectionistic style that can be detail-oriented," she points out.

Honeycutt explains that this drive to do the job correctly means that many responders give 100 percent or more to their work. "Significant others may have a hard time understanding unless someone educates them, that those in our professions are consumed by 'the beast,' " she explains. "The beast is, of course, doing the job well."

Honeycutt emphasizes that a significant other may not understand that an EMS provider feels helpless and wonders: "Was there something I could have done to save my patient's life? Was there one more drug in the drug box I could have given? What if we'd been called sooner?" Or, she explains, the paramedic or firefighter can spend time agonizing over the system by saying "If only the system were better. . . ."

"EMS agencies need to take responsibility for investing in educational programs for significant others of employees," Honeycutt says. "In addition, EMS providers need to have the support of their significant others." She believes that mates need to have knowledge of how intense and how specific the job pressures are. They also need to understand the personality traits of emergency workers.

Honeycutt points out that Employee Assistant Programs aren't always effective in helping responders under stress. "That's because those in emergency work may not feel comfortable talking talking to 'outsiders' about their stress," she says. For example, counselors with limited experience working with EMS providers may have difficulty understanding the full implications of 24-hour shifts and how that impacts a responder.

Significant others, friends, and family members of responders may understand much about EMS stress for the worker. But they don't fully comprehend the reality of running calls. They may even think of it as a glamorous job because they have never been exposed to the reality of it.

There are four specific ways you can help someone—or another can assist you—when stress becomes intense. We have discussed some of these ideas in previous paragraphs, but let's take a look at them again. For example, one person can encourage another person to:

- **Develop a plan of action.** Your mate might say to you, "You certainly have a lot of stress going on. But why not take time to assess what you can change? Is there some kind of action that would help?"

    Every kind of stress must be evaluated to see if there are specific actions that could make a difference. For instance, one coworker can help another reflect in this manner: Could gaining a small piece of new information help? Would talking to someone help? Would making a specific request of some sort help?

    Stress can cause anyone to go around in circles. But the minute a plan of action looks possible, most people feel a little relief. Being able to create a plan of any kind means that one *does* have some control.

- **Develop a plan of coping.** This kind of plan is necessary when there is *nothing you can do to change the initial stress factors.* For instance, if three children have been killed in a car crash, the emergency responder cannot reverse what has happened. But he or she can think about coping measures.

    A helpful plan of coping usually involves a good amount of self-care. If a spouse is under stress, for instance, the other partner can say, "I believe you need to get back into your exercise routine because exercise always helps you feel better."

    A coping plan can also involve adopting a new philosophical viewpoint. One stressed-out person can ask another: "How can you close this out of your mind and move past it? If the shoe were on the other foot here, how would you advise me to move past this dilemma?"

- **Develop a plan of *refocus*.** For instance, if an EMT or paramedic has been hurt by job politics, cumulative stress, or family problems, a plan to *direct attention toward future goals* can help. For instance, if an EMT is becoming burned out on the job, a spouse can say, "How could you refocus your energy so that you'll feel better about yourself? Why don't you focus on two or three things you like about your work? How could you do something positive for your department?"

Reminder

A plan of refocus can help a mate or an EMS partner who is deeply enmeshed in a problem. If you can lead this person to see the importance of making a plan to redirect thinking and personal energy, he or she can get busy designing this plan. You cannot do it for him or her. Your job is to talk about the *importance* of walking down a new path.

- **Develop a plan of renewal.** If someone you care about is in a state of burnout or is feeling very depressed about life in general, a larger plan will be necessary. Focusing on making a few changes, coping, or focusing on new goals *won't be enough*. This person needs encouragement to make a plan for rejuvenating the mind, body, and spirit.

A plan of renewal is really reminding the individual to put deposits back into all of those mental and physical bank accounts that have been depleted. All of the steps don't have to be hard to do or time-consuming, but they do need to be broad-based. For instance, some people might benefit from these steps: Buy a motivational book, commit to an aerobics class twice a week, call an old high school friend, and take two personal leave days. Others might need to do something along these lines: Move to a slightly better neighborhood, design a better self-care program that includes purchasing a hot tub, and make a goal to spend more time out with Mother Nature.

The goal is to design a plan to uplift oneself at the deepest levels of consciousness. This means caring for oneself as a whole person—physically and emotionally. Even if an individual is not particularly religious, there is still a "spiritual" inner self that needs attention. It is that part of the psyche that feels deeply fulfilled and happy *for no particular external reasons*. This part of the self is uplifted by the quality of one's thoughts and how one perceives life. Renewing oneself at the spiritual level requires either connecting to God or somehow feeling a part of the grander scheme of things. This connection to something *outside of oneself* is what lifts the spirit.

FURTHER TIPS

In helping a spouse or significant other under stress, try to create some comforting rituals and small activities that you both enjoy. Make them very simple and easy to implement. Giving each other a back rub, going for a splash in a neighbor's pool, or buying a magazine on cooking that you both enjoy are simple stress relievers. Never overlook small things—from bringing home a potted plant to washing the car—to help your mate feel better.

If the spouse is very stressed out about something in particular, the other partner can ask, "Do you need me to listen? Or would my doing something specific for you help?" For example, a person under stress may not have time to shop for some personal items. Although no one wants to become a full-time gopher or servant to a stressed spouse, doing one or two nurturing things can't hurt.

Try to avoid referring to a spouse or coworker in EMS as "continually stressed-out." This sounds as if that person has a handicap. If you do plan to nurture or help, try to avoid labeling your spouse—or your EMS partner—as "stressed-out all of the time" or "grouchy all of the time." Keep emphasizing that you truly want to help this person feel his or her best—under the present circumstances.

If a coworker is under intense strain, it can help to ask him or her to join you and your family for a meal in a relaxed atmosphere. He or she needs to feel comfort and nurturing in some form. This can be especially hard to attain when one lives alone. Remind anyone under stress to practice self-care by exercising and eating more wisely. Encourage him or her to focus energy on self-nurturing.

When you're not sure of how to help another person under stress, offer to be flexible in the type of help you will give. For instance, if a coworker is having family problems, you might say, "I want you to know that I'm here for you. Tell me how I can help. Would you like me to go somewhere with you? Or, would you like me to just sit quietly and listen? I want to help in any way that would help you to feel better."

If a spouse, friend, or coworker experiences stress over a prolonged period of time, remember to help him or her develop a plan of action, a plan of coping, or a plan of refocus that does not depend too much on the cooperation of others. Remind that person that a plan of renewal means designing self-help. After all, you don't want to create a dependency on you by being *too available*. Remember to give of yourself, but then encourage the other person to become involved in his or her own stress management program.

When it comes to helping an EMS worker who has been through a terrible ordeal at a scene, a spouse or friend can help him or her assess the situation. The following questions may not elicit spoken answers—only thought-provoking introspection. But gently remind the individual that asking the right questions can help bring some closure:

1. Are you satisfied with your performance skills at the scene? Why or why not?
2. Do you have unanswered questions about the scene? Are there bits of information you might seek to help you obtain closure?
3. Are you satisfied with how your coworkers assisted at the scene? Do you feel comfortable that all of you worked well as a team?
4. During the ordeal, what did you learn about medical skills? Did you learn anything that will help you with future calls?
5. Is there anything for which you have to be thankful? Have any good things come from this?
6. How will you refocus your energy? What new challenge might pull your talents in a new direction so you can move past this experience?

Sometimes, individuals can lend great support to others just by acting concerned. Great words of wisdom aren't really necessary. Your attitude of caring toward the other person is what gives the emotional support. Your presence and your emotional availability to your mate, friend, or EMS partner will boost him or her during the tough times.

Being married to an emergency responder, law enforcement officer, or fire-fighter can be very challenging. It is hard to understand why someone pulls into a protective shell—refusing to talk or openly interact—because of a killer day. It can make the spouse feel that he or she is to blame or feel rejected and abandoned. Giving too much love and understanding to a spouse can become draining, especially if no one is giving to the one doing the comforting.

Responders can use touch, eye contact, and writing little notes of appreciation to give something back. "On my darkest days, I can't force a smile sometimes," says Nate, a first responder who works in a challenging urban area. "But I do write little notes for my wife. I can be hilarious in a note. I can be loving and sweet, although I feel mean and edgy. These notes make her feel good, and they take 30 seconds to write. Emergency workers can't forget that spouses need attention."

Reminder

Spouses of emergency workers need to remember that their needs count, too. They need to require their mates to give. This attention may be something as small as 10 minutes of hug time or help in hanging a picture. If giving isn't required—even from a stressed-out mate—anger may build until it explodes internally, or perhaps externally.

Someone who requires no giving is requiring no respect. However, a supportive spouse can try to make the giving easy to do for the spouse under the most stress. After all, each spouse should help the other succeed—even if their roles are not quite equal or balanced at a given time.

YOUR MOST BASIC RELATIONSHIP

As you learn more about relationships in general, remember one obvious fact: The most basic and important relationship we can have is the one we have with ourselves. When we have a good feeling about who we are, we have a good *starting point* for making all of our other relationships work. By having solid self-esteem, we can navigate better within other relationships, including our intimate ones with a spouse or significant other.

If you like yourself as an individual, you can stop reacting so much to others, too. It is easy to read criticism into remarks from others when we don't feel we are doing our best. It is easy to feel unloved when we don't feel we have earned the right to be respected by others. These feelings can sometimes come from how we feel about our past. Whether a bad childhood or a bad former marriage has hurt you, it is important to deal with past issues. *How you view your past has great impact on how bright your future will be.*

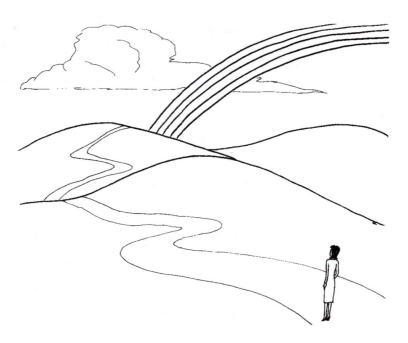

If you don't feel good about past episodes in your life, there are very specific things you can do in order to deal with them. By addressing the past, you can help your present relationships work better. After all, it is very easy to drag past "emotional baggage" into all of your present relationships. When you can feel better about your history, you will feel empowered to support others and care for them. Your self-esteem will be much higher, so that you instinctively act and think in ways that are good for you. Your sense of self-worth will affect everything else that you do.

Reframing

"I'm now convinced that's it's how we view our past that makes or breaks our future," says Suzzan, a clinical psychologist who works with police, fire, and EMS personnel in addition to other patients. *"I often use a method of dealing with the past called reframing to help my clients. Emergency responders sometimes do have a lot of bad issues they need to get over. Like most of the population, most EMTs and paramedics didn't grow up in ideal homes. I'm working with three patients now who are actively trying to reframe their past."*

She continues, *"Think of reframing as an exercise in which you mentally revisit the past. Your goal is to ask, What good came from this which can help me now? The more painful your past is, the more important it is for you to do this. Remember, there is no past so terrible that you cannot learn from it. Reframing a difficult past this way helps you see that all is not lost."*

Suzzan believes that by focusing on the lessons you've learned, the positive insight gained, and the good things accomplished in past battles, you will have tools for improving your life now. A new perspective can't totally erase the pain. But it can help to *neutralize it.*

Coping with a hurtful past can be a challenge for anyone. It's tough to get over problems that have left you angry, confused, sad, hurt, and hopeless. How can you rise above the pain? How can you get on with your life?

> *Whether your past is painful because of abuse, lost love, or financial troubles, you can help yourself heal by "reframing" your loss. Rosemary, who divorced five years ago after her husband left her for another women, says: "I had a turning point in viewing my past. After a couple of years of wallowing around in misery, I decided I did want to feel good about myself. I told myself, 'I can choose how I think and feel about the past and the present.' "*
>
> *She continues, "I journeyed back to the past looking for what was right, what felt good, and what I had accomplished." Reframing helped her let go of her ex-husband's betrayal. She explains: "I saw my former married life as a broader experience than just being with one man. My marriage included some wonderful experiences. Also, I made great friends through my ex. These friends are still in my life. I even obtained a solid business education from working with my ex-husband. He taught me more about running a business than I could have learned anywhere. I have a terrific job as a business consultant today because of being married to him."*

Many psychologists use the method of reframing to help their patients in counseling. Reframing is not denial of anything negative. In fact, totally forgetting terrible pain is probably not humanly possible. Also, reframing is not a substitute for counseling. Reframing won't take the place of grieving or working though the initial shock of bad issues such as divorce, abuse, or betrayal. *But it can help you recover faster.* Reframing is a way to *obtain closure.* When you reframe your past relationships that have caused you pain, you will be in a much better position to have healthy, productive relationships now.

> *Trying to deny a real tragedy or loss can be self-destructive. So focusing on your past in a new way should only be done after lots of soul searching. It is important to deal with parts of it which were hurtful. But then try to reframe your past in a way that spells hope, not despair. This is an excellent way to improve the likelihood that you will have a more positive future. When your future looks brighter, you will attract more positive and upbeat people into your life, too.*

Revisiting your past will take time and effort. Try these suggestions for taking another look at your personal history:

- **First get in a positive frame of mind.** If you reframe when you are in a bad mood, you'll have a tougher time succeeding. Don't try to reframe when you are tired. Your brain won't access the healthiest information.

- **Realize that only the upbeat will empower you.** No one has ever been empowered by negative thoughts. Feeling mean and angry can give you an adrenaline rush. But this craziness will eventually *land you against a brick wall.* You will feel stuck at a bad point in your life, and you won't be able to get past it.

  For example, Jenny, a divorced single mother, used to fantasize about physically hurting her ex-husband. "Those imaginary beatings I gave him made me feel good for a while," laughs Jenny. "But these daily rehearsals of tar-and-feathering were just wasted energy. I knew I had to empower myself with healthier thoughts. I started dwelling on all the good I had ever experienced. I drew a better picture of my past and present. That's how you flush a lot of bad memories down the drain."

- **Make a written list of the good you gained in your past.** Make the list as long as possible. By seeing good thoughts on paper about positive aspects of your trying experience, you will feel that your gains *truly were real, not wishful dreaming.* Turn it into a project. Invest a solid amount of time in reframing. By writing things down, you can come back later to reflect on each point.

Codependency

As you work to improve the relationships in your life, keep in mind that many EMS professionals—not to mention nurses, doctors, firefighters, and police personnel—are codependent. This simply means that they have a tendency to *over*-function, *over* work, and *over* help in a lot of situations. They feel overly responsible when it comes to taking care of others. This can be good in a sense, because our society needs people who will look out for others. However, you want to *help others appropriately*—not participate in life in such a way that you are draining yourself.

Mary Ann Kane, Ed.D., a psychologist and director of counseling services at Notre Dame College in Manchester, New Hampshire, says: "Not all codependents are pulled into someone else's problems. A codependent will just as quickly *pull in* somebody to act out codependency with. Codependents often grow up in a household where a parent was a substance abuser or exhibited out-of-control behaviors. They feel in control when they encourage others to lean on them."

Dr. Kane believes that excessive caretaking of others is a personality trait developed out of the need to survive a chaotic childhood. Taking care of children, sick patients, or the elderly is *not* codependency. Being overly responsible for mature adults who should be working to fix their own problems is. For example, if you find yourself worrying too much over a coworker, brother, friend, or patient who clearly has out-of-control behaviors, it can be easy to get pulled into playing almost a "parental" role to this individual.

However, having to do too much for another person—when he or she is not trying to recover from the problem at all—is not fair to you. Sooner or later, you will wake up to find that a dependent person's problems have exhausted you. All of your "helping" didn't help a thing.

Caretaking another person's life or emotions never works anyway. Out-of-control people will resist our efforts—even double or triple their stubbornness—to *prove* we can't control them. Subsequently, they become experts at manipulation. The dependent person with a compulsive disorder, for example, is *already* being controlled by alcohol, gambling, food, sex, or drugs. Why would he or she want to be controlled by a person also?

"A closer look at trying to 'fix' someone reveals a fairly simple fact," says Dr. Kane. "This caretaking requires the belief that the one you're helping is incompetent. Caretaking means doing for someone what he or she should be doing."

> *"I was always trying to help my alcoholic brother," says Rita, a paramedic from the South. "I was very codependent. I had to learn to draw the line on what I would or would not do for him. I do call to check on how he's doing. He knows I love him very much. But I don't lend him money or support his drinking problem. I gave him my bottom line on his problems. I told him, "I will do anything I can to help you, but I won't do anything to hurt myself."*

There are many excellent books on codependency issues in the self-help section of bookstores. If you believe that you are in a relationship with a person who is out-of-control concerning alcoholism or certain behaviors, it would benefit you to read more about codependency—which is a very complex issue. But once you identify whether you fit the true definition of what a codependent is, it's easier to start taking better care of yourself. You will need to follow a recovery program yourself. It will take time and effort to stop trying to control others.

There are many definitions of what codependency is. If you find yourself taking up too much slack for someone *on a regular basis,* you may very well be codependent. However, learning to deal with codependency will help you to prevent job burnout in EMS. You will gradually learn *how much to give* and still feel good about yourself. Your talents and skills must be utilized appropriately, or you will use up much-needed energy that should be used to keep your own ship afloat.

Sharing job info with your children

Your relationship with each of your children can be difficult to maintain when job pressures impact you. Perhaps you wonder if you should share more about your work stress with a child, so that he or she can comprehend why you are in a bad mood. Or, would that be too much for a child to handle? It is hard to be under a lot of pressure without your family knowing what is going on. You need to figure out how much to tell them.

Children can't learn coping skills if adults always pretend everything's fine. Children need to see you confront problems, cope as best you can, and bounce back. Still, although your children need to understand the basics of what you do—how you help save lives or property, some of the dangers involved, and the importance of your work—they should not be told gruesome details. Even if you're trying to impress upon your 17-year-old the dangers of driving too fast, do not share with him or her the details of the accident you recently worked. Children need protection from too much pain, and there is definitely a limit on what you should reveal about EMS to them.

It is a good idea to take your children to work with you occasionally. Let them talk with your coworkers. Assign them some simple tasks, such as sharpening pencils or stacking papers. Acquaint them with the equipment your department uses and let them tour the vehicles. You might also drive them to the hospital to show them where you take your patients for further care. Children do need to have a mental image of where you work.

One reason children need to see your work environment is that they are actually reassured about your safety when they can picture you on the job. They need to know, however, that real emergency work is not always so glamorous or so neatly packaged as TV shows portray. They also need to understand that true emergencies don't always have satisfying conclusions and that this is partially the reason for a lot of your stress.

Help your children see that your work involves getting to a scene quickly, racing against the clock, and facing situations that may be raging out of control—just like on TV. But also share with them: "Unlike on TV, sometimes what is out of control can't be fixed. People do die, and houses do get destroyed by fire." Explain to them that your own stress levels skyrocket when you lose the control that you were striving to achieve at a scene.

Your relationship with your child should involve a lot of honesty about how vulnerable a tough job can make you feel. Tell your child openly when you are bent out of shape because of work. If you try to avoid this honesty, children may think you're angry with them if you show a lack of patience. When you are under a lot of stress, you may either clam up or talk too much. Explain to your children that this is the way stressed individuals behave, but try not to act out your moods excessively in front of them.

The best way to allay a child's fears about the dangers of your work is to emphasize your preparation for the job. Talk about the study and rigorous training emergency work mandates. Find out how much your kids really know about what it takes to do your job well. When you gain insight into your children's understanding, you can then paint a broader, more accurate picture of your skills.

If you are a firefighter, there's nothing wrong with telling your children that you do get a chance to be a hero, daredevil, champion, and lifesaver. But also point out to each child why the job requires skills in math, physics, mechanics, and good communication. Don't forget to mention the abilities your job requires for staying cool under pressure and getting along with other people.

Also, explain to your children that they personally can help save lives. They can give help, solicit help, relay information, and soothe and calm others during an emergency. Every child should know lifesaving skills, fire prevention tips, and how to spot trouble that could lead to disaster. Stress to your offspring that children can be primary troubleshooters. They can spot fire hazards, poisonous materials, and potentially dangerous scenarios just as quickly as adults can.

In addition, excellent safety training manuals for children are available through the American Red Cross. These manuals contain entertaining stories, games, and artwork pertaining to water safety, fire prevention, safe ways to be home alone, how to dial 911 with correct information, what to do when someone is poisoned, how to report suspicious adults who might harm children, and dozens more incidents a child might encounter.

Although you don't want to dwell on accidents or emergency response too much with your children, helping them to feel a part of your work in some way will create a bond with them about your chosen profession. Naturally, you want your children to feel that your work is important to the community. This way, if you do have to work Christmas Eve, they can better understand the importance of your sacrifice.

Job stress and family life

If you are having trouble keeping connected with your family due to job stress, remember that you must find ways to make it all work. The following tips can help you keep your family together during stressful times:

- **Create dependability.** Make a two-minute call during certain times of the day. When you tell a child or spouse, "I'll do my best to call between five and six o'clock every day," this gives them something to count on. Children, especially, thrive on *predictability*.
- **Find common ground.** For example, everyone can watch the same video during the week—even if everyone watches at different times. Then over the weekend, discuss the video at a sit-down meal.

- **Require family teamwork.** Divide chores into small parts. For example, in doing the laundry, a six-year-old can carry baskets of folded clothes to the bedroom. An older child can be responsible for putting shirts on hangers. A family that works together develops a sense of closeness and pride about belonging to the family.
- **Stay plugged into each other.** Post everyone's schedule in full view. By knowing everyone's whereabouts, you'll feel connected. Conflicts can also be resolved before they get out of hand when schedules are posted. If one child needs to be at piano practice, another child may need to make other arrangements about attending a birthday party.
- **Create small rituals that help you feel bonded as a family.** For example, at bedtime you can do a simple "10 hugs and 10 kisses" if you are too tired to read a story. Children love rituals, and rituals stick fondly in a child's memory forever.

How you manage your part in personal and professional relationships is a very involved and ongoing process. No matter how hard you try, your relationships will never be stress-free. All human relationships are complex and flawed. But when you see that making mistakes is all part of the growth process in any relationship, you can relax and enjoy each relationship more. In fact, you can only enjoy relationships when you do not expect perfection from them.

REVIEW ACTIVITIES

1. What are two ways you can set a verbal boundary with another person?
2. Why do well-placed boundaries keep relationships healthy?
3. What is the "policy of joint agreement" in marriage?
4. Why is a relationship not healthy if you can't give it a bottom line on how you will participate?
5. List three reasons why becoming codependent is destructive to the one who does excessive caretaking of others.
6. Name two characteristics of a destructive relationship between dating partners.
7. How can a busy parent create dependability and predictability for a child?
8. Name three ways a busy family can stay connected through shared activities.

For Supervisors

1. Let's say that one of your employees is angry a good deal of the time. He or she is having emotional outbursts. How might you address this situation with this individual? How could you offer sympathy and support but still require this person to deal with the issue?

2. You've learned that one of your personnel is having marital problems. These problems are affecting his or her work performance. How might you assist this individual without prying into his or her private life? Do you know of any good relationship tapes or videos to recommend to this individual? Do you know of a chaplain or other professional who could offer support?

3. A possible project: As a supervisor, make it a point to keep files of contact names of counselors, chaplains, and social workers who might help stressed individuals. Also, try starting a file of good book titles, video titles, and magazine clippings on self-help topics and family–marital issues for your staff to utilize.

Class Projects

1. Plan a hypothetical seminar on family and work stress. What issues should be addressed in this seminar regarding EMS–public safety work and how it impacts family life? Name individuals in your community who might help organize such a project.

2. Name at least five ways that an EMS department can offer emotional support to the family members of workers. For example, would a station "support group" that meets once a month help? Would a department newsletter featuring employees' tips for lowering stress be a good idea?

CHAPTER SEVEN

TIME AND MONEY MANAGEMENT– ORGANIZATIONAL SKILLS

Whether your career goal is to climb to top levels of management in EMS, or you want to continue working happily as an EMT until you retire, it helps to manage your time and money well. This all starts by being an organized individual who can manage *all* available resources with a good measure of expertise, both at work and at home.

"I was almost fired when I was a young paramedic," confides Harry, who now owns one-fourth of a large, private ambulance service. "I made some serious mistakes on the job during my first year. I won't bore you with the details, but I was all shook up over splitting up with my girlfriend, so I was very distracted. Well, I resolved to make myself more valuable to the company before my boss threw me out on the pavement. I started helping him in every way I could think of.

"This small ambulance service where I worked was a shaky business. The budget was so pitiful we'd have payroll checks bounce from time-to-time. But I wanted to work there, so I decided I'd become a bona fide expert on efficiency. I helped the boss pinch pennies in the right places. I offered suggestions for cutting response time on calls. I worked overtime to prove I was a team player."

He continues, "I absolutely loved being a paramedic, and I knew I had to prove myself as a reliable person after nearly getting the ax. I started learning the business inside and out. I visited other stations on my days off, learning everything I could. I kept notes on how other responders were saving money and improving service. I read every bit of information on time management and getting organized that I could find.

"I organized the supply room, polished the ambulances, cleaned the bathrooms, and made myself into something of a general pain, I'm sure," he laughs. "But I swear this early fear of losing my job is probably the very reason I own part of this business today. I had to carve myself a niche, so I learned to manage resources. Managing time and money well will practically guarantee that you're going to be a success in life."

Having good skills for managing resources—and figuring out how to improvise well if you don't have an abundance of them—will help you to reach your goals. If you can't manage time and money well, you are going to feel extremely frustrated. You will probably wonder, "Am I on the wrong career track?"

If you eventually decide you want a different job in EMS or a different career altogether, that's fine. Your basic training as an emergency responder is a solid career foundation. But whatever happens to you along the road of life will be more under your direct control if you figure out how to become an efficient individual. You can do that if you learn to use your time, money, and other resources for your maximum benefit.

You don't have to become obsessive about time or money. After all, you don't want to become so frugal that you can't spend a cent without feeling guilty. You also don't want to become so driven by the clock that you can't enjoy a golden sunset. But you do want to gain a reasonable amount of control in managing all of your resources, *so that your stress levels will go down.*

By evaluating what you are already doing—and facing squarely up to what you need to improve upon—you can reach your goals and hold stress at bay. In addition, if you become adept at making improvements in scheduling and getting organized, you will learn to feel more confident if you decide to become a supervisor or manager in EMS.

WHAT TIME OPTIONS ARE AVAILABLE?

Time is a fixed thing, of course. Although you cannot control the clock or stretch time in any sense of the word, you can manage yourself in relation to it. It helps to think of time management as *personal energy management.* You can manage your responsibilities in ways that help you stop wasting vital energy that could be put to better use. What helps is to think of time management as somewhat of a game. That game is to find out how much control you can take back from the clock. Then use that time to reduce your stress levels.

Time saved each day should ideally be spent with people you love or doing things you love. A little more freedom to spend time in an enjoyable way will put balance back into your life. Without a decent moment of healthy "down time," you are cutting deeply into your emotional well-being. But what are most people tempted to do with small amounts of time they save? They fill the time slots right back up, and *they're still on a treadmill!*

Reminder

In time management, you can implement as few or as many time-savers as you wish. You can find your cutoff point wherever it feels right to you. But if you learn just one or two good time-saving skills, you will probably want to try more.

Your strategy should be:

- Find one new thing that saves you just five or ten minutes of time.
- Stick with your time-saver *until it becomes a habit.*
- Implement additional time-saving strategies until you feel more in control.

"One of the best time management tricks I've learned is to group similar tasks together whenever possible," says Donna, a first responder. *"I used to have an extremely hard time managing my job and my family. But when I started to get more organized, I figured out that I should plan all errands together. Likewise, I'll sit down and make five phone calls at once. Plus, I'll make out meal plans for one month at a time."*

She continues, *"If it's at all possible, I try to deal with personal items I need to purchase for my family in one day. I work from lists and plan my stops. I used to zigzag all over town on my days off. I couldn't accomplish anything, and I'd wind up with nothing done and a bad headache."*

These strategies can help you think about saving more *personal energy*—and therefore more time—either in your work role or in your personal life:

- **Always work from a master list.** Instead of having scraps of paper and sticky notes all over the place, keep a thick composition notebook with you at all times. Write your "to-do" list in large clear letters, even if it stretches for several pages. Then from this list, create an "action list" for each day.
- **Set priorities to focus your energy.** If you can't figure out what is really important to accomplish at any given moment, you will constantly feel torn. This torn feeling will drain your batteries. Practice identifying your most important goals for each day to avoid getting sidetracked with unimportant phone calls and other time wasters.

- **Make a plan for every true goal.** A plan can be as simple as two or three steps. But with no plan at all, you're likely to skip over things you really would like to do. For instance, if you want to exercise three times a week, you have to figure out how to make that happen. Your plan might be telling yourself this: "I'll work out on my days off between two and three o'clock."

- **Don't underestimate how long a job will take.** Be realistic about how much time everything requires, so that you can complete your daily plans. Your goal in life should not be to accomplish every activity that sounds inviting. You can't. No one has that kind of energy. You goal should be to choose what is really important.

  Try to spend enough time on each project, so that you feel you are doing a good job. By allowing enough time to complete assignments or chores, you will create a series of successes in your life. This will reduce your stress, because you will feel in control of the clock—not the other way around.

- **Don't forget to "steal" some transitional time.** Everyone needs time to calm down, get refocused, and let tension subside. Without this time to change gears, you will feel very stressed. You probably will be tempted to skip your exercise or other self-care needs in order to keep pushing to beat the clock. Take time to pause and let some energy flow back into your psyche.

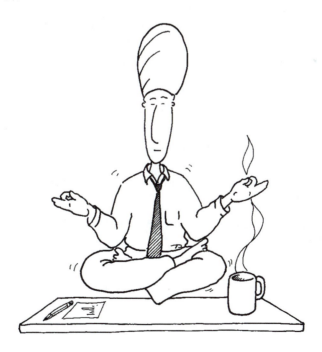

Although good time-savers put slack in the rope, so to speak, there are also "time-bending" concepts that help you manipulate your schedule to balance work and family.

Concepts such as the following will get you on track for thinking up more on your own:

- **Make time deposits ahead of schedule.** For example, if holiday emergencies might keep you from your child's school play, visit the classroom in advance to watch rehearsals, offer refreshments, or help with costumes. Even if you stay only 45 minutes, your child will feel your involvement.

  If you can't show up on the big night, have someone videotape your child's performance. Watch it later with your child.

  Another good idea: If your mate craves a special night out on the town once a month, take him or her out the week *before* training sessions cram your schedule.

- **Think minutes, not hours.** It's those small but frequent acts of kindness you do that keep you bonded with family members. Five-second hugs can't make up for longer special times together, but frequency of contact goes a long way in keeping you emotionally plugged in with a spouse or child.

  Place one-minute "I miss you" calls to your mate or bring home your teenager's favorite ice cream when your day is hectic. This says, "I'm busy, but your needs are important to me."

- **Double the fun on time slots.** When you spend time away from home with your spouse or significant other—whether it's one hour or three—try to fit in errands or activities you both want to do. That way each of you will feel more *emotionally satisfied* within the time allotted.

  For example, if you want your husband to help you buy paint for the kitchen, offer to let him choose the restaurant for lunch. Or, encourage him to choose an activity or errand that is important to him.

✔ Take control of as many aspects of your life as you can on the job and at home.

For example, families will feel less stressed if they draw up daily to-do lists and charts of who does what. This kind of planning is the key to finding more quality time. Children who learn to pull some of their own weight on maintaining the family routine will feel more confident and emotionally grounded.

*Let's look at a great way to organize a family of four
on tackling chores:*

Give each person *two* 10-minute chores to accomplish per day. Write the exact chores under each name. Post them on the refrigerator door where they can't be overlooked. Let's say that vacuuming the family room takes 10 minutes. Let's call throwing in a load of laundry a 10-minute chore. Cleaning a bathtub could be called a 10-minute chore, give or take a minute or two. Label all chores that will reasonably fit this category—washing out a garbage can or cleaning a toilet—as 10-minute tasks.

If four people do two 10-minute tasks per day, that's eight chores or 80 minutes worth of chores per day. Yes, it's acceptable to do two or three days' worth of chores together as long as they get done. In a 30-day month, four people can accomplish a total of 2,400 minutes of chores—or 40 hours of housework! Because these were *focused* 10-minute segments of work, that's 40 *solid* hours of "nonstop" cleaning. This is what family teamwork can do. Explain to your family how much your collective efforts can accomplish. Track your chores for two months. Your house should be clean, if not spotless.

Although this kind of teamwork is productive for a family, it can also benefit your EMS station. Being neat and orderly within an environment requires *the input of all who live or work there.* "Well," you might say, "I don't see why I should care about great organizational skills, tidiness, or spiffing up the station. I don't own the ambulance company I work for. I'm not the top dog who's going to be held accountable if everything is not shipshape."

The answer to that is this: Having these skills will make you more valuable to your employer. It is impossible to *not* be noticed for having good organizational skills. They will become part of your persona. Everything from your effectiveness on the job to your personal appearance will reflect it. When you become an efficient person who pitches in to making your division run smoother, your boss would be foolish *not* to put you in the highest position available for your skills when that position become open.

At least if layoffs ever occur, you're going to be one of the last people your boss would want to let go. You will have earned a spot in the company success plan if you can arrange things well; organize equipment, supplies, and schedules; and maintain tidiness in every form. *You're a superachiever if you can help others do the same.*

Pulling your act together

If you have ever been around superachievers, you probably have figured out pretty quickly that they usually are very organized. Of course, getting organized is synonymous with managing time better. No one can accomplish a great deal in *any* profession, nor in his or her personal life, without getting organized. It all starts with being as neat and orderly as possible.

Creating a neat environment is a habit worth acquiring. You can learn to stay on top of things by constantly creating neatness, instead of chaos, all around you. Your creating a neat environment, at work or home, requires *creating lots of small systems* that will support your efforts. A well-organized environment will help you accomplish your tasks with less stress. A neat environment, from your sock drawer to your station's equipment storage room, will help you save time and energy in the long run.

For example: Clutter is a stressful reminder that constantly tells you that *you have put off making decisions.* Rather than deal with the junk in your attic or your living area, you've pushed it aside. Having too much clutter around you is proof that you have failed to take action. This in itself will make you feel out of control.

> *"A couple of years ago, I almost fainted when I looked into my car trunk before a summer vacation," laughs Carl, a paramedic instructor. "I had in there, among the junk, a fairly expensive Christmas present I'd forgotten to wrap. It was a necklace for my wife.*
>
> *"My bad habits still haven't improved," he declares. "Not long ago, I opened my trunk one afternoon to discover a bag of groceries I'd forgotten about from the night before. Yes, you guessed it. There were milk and eggs in the bag. I swear I'm fairly organized in my work life, but my personal life is very disorganized."*

If you are out of practice, your getting into the full swing of becoming more organized will feel awkward at first. It takes a concerted effort to change bad habits. But stick with the process. You're training your brain to help you manage time. With that time saved, you can either conquer your goals or find time to have more fun.

The following list will help you think about how to manage yourself, so that you can save time. There is nothing new here. You've heard it all before. You probably learned it all in kindergarten. But sometimes, we need to be reminded of why something works. When you become very busy, it is tempting to toss aside the rules you do know because of pressing problems of the moment. But review these suggestions to see where you might begin to *practice* getting organized:

- **Avoid backtracking.** When you begin a task, try to follow through to the end. Be very big on closure. Of course, this isn't always possible, but when it is, train yourself to stick with bringing a task to full completion. The time it takes to start up a project again, once you've dropped it, is enormous.
- **Do have a place for everything.** We have all heard the old adage of staying organized: "Have a place for everything and keep everything in its place." Well, it still is excellent advice. The time you spend looking for items is time that you don't have as a busy person.

You must create places for your possessions by finding or buying drawers, shelves, cabinets, baskets, dividers, folders, storage bins. Don't beat yourself up for having a mess on your hands. Maybe the stuff around you does not have a "home." Get busy designating a home for everything from your keys to your favorite reference books.

At work, if your budget does not allow for new purchases, do everything you can to get organizational tools donated to your department. Employees can feel out of control working in a station or small substation where clutter abounds.

- **Use labels abundantly.** For example, use clearly printed labels with large lettering for stored boxes of equipment. This can save hours of searching for items at work. Also, labeling and dating food in your station's freezer or refrigerator can help things run smoother. How many times have you tossed out something because you weren't sure of when it was purchased?

Regarding labeling, don't forget to improve your filing system whenever possible. One trick is to have clearly printed "guide sheets" in the front of each file cabinet drawer to help you locate needed information. The guide sheet should tell you which files are *within* a drawer.

Clearly labeling every diskette for your computer system is crucial for saving time, too. Skipping the labeling process, or labeling poorly, can cost you hours of work when you can't locate needed documents at home or in your EMS office.

Start small, but begin somewhere . . .

Here's an example of how one good decision to get organized could save you lots of time and stress:

"When I first got promoted to a supervisor's job years ago, I was really a mess on paperwork," says Richard, a fire chief from Idaho. "I was trying to clip and read articles from professional journals, so this made messy stacks of papers. Also, I was dealing with the paperwork for two committees I served on. Then I had papers I wanted to keep related to educational grants for employees. My cubbyhole at the station was a fire hazard—no pun intended."

He continues, "This older man who volunteered at our division finally showed me how to use colored folders to sort things out. Now, this is going to sound simple, but sometimes simple is all you need. I now use a red folder to hold papers marked 'urgent business.' My green folder is for items to be read at leisure; blue is for phone calls I should make within two or three weeks, and so forth.

"I've learned to color-code everything—even rows of personal lockers for our fire-fighters who need to get quickly equipped for a call. I put red stickers on certain

file drawers with urgent business. At home, I use large red packets for bills that need paying and tax papers that need quick attention. I'm still messy in a lot of ways, but I do get the big stuff done."

By spending just a few dollars on folders, you can save yourself countless time on rummaging around for what you need. If you are a new supervisor in EMS, you might want to get started on color coding paperwork and other business. The following list for color coding is one that a lot of managers now use:

- The red folders will hold your urgent items (bills that must be paid quickly, deadlines to meet, VIP calls to return).
- Blue folders will contain nonurgent calls to return (a civic group needing a speaker in the next three months, a travel agency you wanted to contact).
- Orange will hold your to-do lists and action items (inspections to conduct, a new résumé to review).
- The green folders will hold your "review" items (materials for upcoming EMS conferences, new equipment you'd like to budget for).

It is important to remember that most tips for getting organized must be simple or they're probably not going to work over a period of time. Naturally, taking a computer course to learn new software programs for creating efficiency in your department is not exactly simple. Neither is taking a three-day seminar on time management skills. But for the most part, any habit or change you implement personally must be relatively easy to do, or it will end up costing you time.

Of course, organizing your daily planner or figuring out your calendar a year in advance—as many EMS professionals do—takes a lot of focus. But the concepts of keeping track of events and time slots must be relatively simple. If not, you won't remember *the flow* of those plans you have created.

Think tools to save time

Instead of browbeating yourself about something that is out of control, ask better questions such as: "What change would help? How could I find a viable alternative?" In order to save time, get organized, and neaten a cluttered environment, your buying small "tools" can help fix your problems.

In Chapter 1, Angie, a supervisor of 12 EMTs and paramedics in the Southeast, shared a story about how she got her household clutter under control. She needed to tackle a large accumulation of toys, laundry, newspapers, and junk all over her three-bedroom home. By buying just one small organizational tool each week, she finally got her house looking fine.

Her "tools" were relatively simple for making changes. At first, she bought hooks for hanging more of her children's belongings. Then she bought five cheap laundry baskets for sorting toys and other items. Each week she made a positive move to tackle her situation.

Here are some of the time-saving devices you might want to try:

- **A dry erasable board to post family schedules.** These boards are available in calendar form or as bulletin boards. Debbie Glenn, ambulance director for Fire–EMS in Ellingwood, Kansas, says such a board makes it easy for her husband to know where to find her at any hour of the day. Debbie juggles marriage, motherhood, volunteer work, teaching college, and a host of other activities.

- **A speaker phone.** Jay Fitch, Ph.D., president of Fitch & Associates, an EMS consulting firm based in Kansas City, Missouri, says, "I travel three to five days a week, but I'm at the dinner table with my family every night. We installed a speaker phone in the kitchen. I chat with my wife and children individually, even though I may be in Alaska."

- **An expandable file for personal bills.** You can buy prelabeled expandable folders that have sections for your mortgage, electric bill, phone, car payment, and so forth.

  Have you ever struggled to find an overdue electric bill for your home or apartment? It was not in your basket of bills, it wasn't above the sun visor in your car, and it wasn't on your desk at work. You had to call the electric company to check the amount owed. If you had to drive the payment to a payment center, you probably killed your entire morning on this snafu. With a prelabeled expandable file, you can drop all of your bills into the right sections of the file the minute they come in.

Although you don't want tools or devices that only complicate your life—electric knives that clutter your kitchen or foot massagers you'll never use—the right tools in your home and work environment can relieve stress. For example, many people swear by paying their bills via computer software.

If you saved one hour per week by paying your bills online, you would save 52 hours per year—the equivalent of a full workweek! It is very easy to spend two hours or more each week going through bills, addressing envelopes, writing out checks, and driving across town to the post office. If you don't have a home computer, you should at least buy a book or two of stamps as a "time-saving tool." You can then save time by using a drive-up box at the post office or by mailing your bills from home.

Ask yourself: What will help me save time each and every week?

Reminder

Let's play "what if" for a moment. By getting organized, let's say that you could save:

- An hour each week on doing laundry. For example, by planning wisely, you could wash only full loads, instead of doing several smaller loads.

- An hour every week on cooking. You might prepare casseroles to freeze ahead or designate one night a week "soup and sandwich" night.

- An hour each week on paying bills. For instance, you might go ahead and write checks for all of your unpaid bills on a Sunday afternoon. If you aren't ready to mail them, you could address the envelopes, add stamps, and put them in your expandable file. When your usual mailing date arrives for each bill, you've got each one ready to send.

By saving three hours each week in this manner, you will have saved the equivalent of three full 52-hour workweeks in a year!

More control measures

When you force yourself to slow down and think of ideas for getting everything organized, you will discover ways to change things within your scheduling and your environment to reduce your stress. But having a good idea in front of you won't change a thing. Your *decisions to take action* will improve a situation. In fact, the only way to reduce your stress is to make real decisions. Decisions are easier to make if you feel confident that your planning is on target.

For example, many EMS–fire division managers insist that planning for family time works better if it is done one year in advance. The school calendar, the work calendar, and the community events calendar can all be better coordinated this way. If you decide to try this method of scheduling, think in terms of meeting *emotional needs* in the process.

One fire chief told us he plans time off around dinner theater events, because he and his wife both love to go. Another paramedic says he plans a vacation each year around an antique car show. His two adult sons go with him. Another fire chief told us he plans three separate "weekend minivacations" each year. "I take only one of my three children each time," he explains. "That way I can give that child my full attention."

Many prehospital emergency responders say they involve their families in seminars, travel for work, or community projects sponsored by their employers. You can

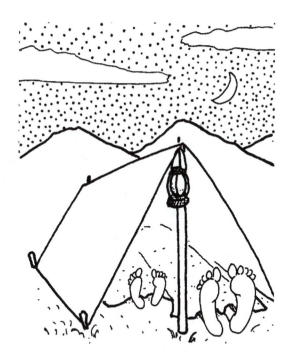

figure out how to do the same if you hold family discussions to identify needs. As we mentioned in Chapter 1, needs are so important that you should *navigate by them.*

By openly talking about everyone's needs, you can all work together in a more harmonious fashion concerning time planning. It is easy to be with family members and still not know their hopes, plans, or dreams.

"Balancing is a day-to-day process," says Mike Nepolitano, fire chief of Great Bend Fire and EMS in Kansas. "It takes great flexibility. But I believe that your family must come before work. You can't neglect your work, but valuing family first puts everything else in perspective."

MONEY MATTERS

While organizing your time and activities, remember to work at organizing your finances also. Learning better money management skills will reduce stress in your life more effectively than almost anything else you can do. Money issues are stressful because they are so connected to *everything.* You can't take your child to the doctor without financial resources, and you can't run your EMS department without cash.

Money is closely related to time management in a lot of ways also. When time is short, it is tempting to spend too much money on fast food or an overpriced gift on a credit card. When the clocking is ticking away, it can be too much trouble to figure out a better way.

Your choices don't necessarily have to be earth shattering. A series of small improvements can improve your financial situation. In addition, remember to *keep* doing those things that are already working well for you. For example, Keith, who holds a management position in a large urban EMS department, has figured out that he should have maintained the money management skills he acquired early in his career.

> *Keith shares this story: "When I was a young EMT, I made thirteen thousand dollars a year. I tried so hard to budget that tiny salary, that I did a really fine job. I actually had a sizable savings account. But now that I'm making forty thousand a year, I'm not as much in control. I have too much debt, and I waste too much money.*
>
> *"I'll buy twenty-five dollars worth of fast food to take home a couple of times a week, because I'm too tired to cook for my kids," he says. " Or, I'll go to the automotive section of a store when I'm in a big hurry. And I'll end up charging the most expensive tires they sell."*
>
> *He continues, "I need to be a lot more careful, so I'll have something when I retire. Like most of my busy friends, I spend money for fast food as a way of saving time. I've gotten kind of lazy about budgeting because I'm constantly on the go. But if I'd go back to the thriftiness of my young EMT years, I'd have a lot more to show for my efforts."*

When you're not happy with the way you're budgeting, either in your department or in your home life, it is important to assess carefully what's going on. Like Keith, who managed more wisely when his budget was tight, you can simply neglect to use the financial management skills you already possess. It can be hard to find time to keep track of income, expenses, and all the paperwork that Uncle Sam or local governments demand. However, carving out "thinking time" and planning sessions for yourself is imperative.

Practice makes perfect

Think about money management this way: Why not turn earning, spending, saving, and investing money into a challenge you enjoy getting control of? Any task in life is easier to accomplish if you have a little passion for seeing results. Money skills can be sharpened in ways similar to those in time management. For example, try to master a few concepts about saving money, turn each change into a habit, and then master a few more strategies.

Even if your salary is very small, it still is important to learn all you can about money management. Read articles on financial matters and borrow good investment books from your public library. Study investing carefully, even if you haven't a dime to invest. By the time you do have more funds, you want to be ready to act. Three years from now, you could be earning a larger salary. Or, your spouse might be earning more. A relative or friend could leave you some cash in a will. You might be working at a larger station, or you could get a promotion with a salary increase. When your salary does rise, or if your financial picture improves in some fashion, you want to be prepared to take advantage of putting any extra money to better use.

The following are financial questions deemed important by several young EMTs and firefighters across the country. The answers will help you to comprehend some of the basic concepts of financial planning. Reflect on the answers in order to find one or two approaches for helping your own financial picture.

1. Is it worth the trouble to save only a small amount of money each month? For example, if I can save only $25 per month, isn't that too insignificant to matter?
    Answer: Remember that small amounts do add up over time. For example, figure up how much you would have in the bank if you had saved $25 per month since your fifteenth birthday. If you are 30 now, you would have over $6,700 if your money, compounded monthly, had earned 5 percent interest. *Patience is the key to watching money grow.*

2. What should be my main goal concerning money? Should I concentrate on making more of it, saving it, or learning to invest it?
    Answer: Ideally you want to do all three. However, your chief goal over the long term should be *to build net worth.* For example, if you have $5,000 in assets, but you owe $2,000 in debts, your net worth is $3,000. A person who owns a $100,000 house with a $90,000 mortgage against it has a net worth of $10,000.

3. How do some people manage so well financially? Do they have some magic touch I failed to inherit?
    Answer: If you know people who are great with money, they understand a simple principle. They know how to "live below" their means. They work at scrimping so they will have cash to invest. This cash could be a down payment on a house or land. Or, it could be invested in stocks or bonds. They know better than to spend more than they make.

4. I'm worried about my spending habits. I buy things I can't afford, and I do a lot of financial juggling. Is it really bad to "live it to the max"?
    Answer: If you are worried about your spending habits, it is wise to be concerned. Let this be your wake-up call. If you *consistently* spend more than you make, eventually you will go *broke.* If you have a major problem such as an extended illness or job loss, you almost certainly will have to declare bankruptcy. You can curtail this in two ways: Reduce your spending or increase your income. We discuss more about this below.

5. Are credit cards all bad? On my salary, I sure can't pay cash all of the time.

    Answer: Credit cards are not all bad if you buy needed items at 25 percent or more savings. Then pay the balance off each month. Your credit rating will look fine and you will offset the cost of the card's annual fee if you locate bargains. Concentrate on charging items you would have to buy at full price anyway.

6. How can I keep track of all the bills, bank statements, and IRS-related material? My finances are a jumbled-up mess of paperwork.

    Answer: If your financial papers are in disarray, buy file folders. Separate all bills, insurance papers, and other related money info into 10 to 20 different folders. As mentioned in the time-saving tips of this chapter, a prelabeled expandable folder for basic bills (housing, telephone, utilities, life insurance) works well. Organizing your paperwork with folders makes it easier to keep receipts for Uncle Sam.

7. I've decided I would like to save money every month in a savings account. I've read that you should pay yourself first. Many times I have started, then quit. How can I be sure I'll have it to save?

    Answer: To discipline yourself to save money, start with an extremely reasonable small amount. The amount is not as important as the savings *habit* you're developing. Save the same amount every month. If you can boost the amount later, start another *separate* savings account. Then later, as you keep up this discipline, start another account. You eventually will get a *feel* for how to manage your savings. However you choose to save, never stop saving that original amount in your *first account* no matter how you have to scrimp.

8. I want to be a millionaire someday. Am I dreaming too big?

    Answer: Most millionaires do not become millionaires until they pass 60 years of age. Younger millionaires are the *exception* to the rule. If you are a young EMT with a good measure of foresight and discipline, becoming a millionaire is not that far-fetched.

    If you are 20 years old, and you saved just $60 a month—getting 11.5 percent interest, compounded monthly (which is very doable in certain investment plans), and letting the money roll over until you're 65—you would have a million dollars. So, yes, even a young EMT can someday attain millionaire status.

All individuals develop a personal money management style. No two people perceive money issues exactly alike. By educating yourself, you will learn which concepts will serve you and your budget well.

Here are a few quick lessons on personal money matters:

- **Do you actively look for value?** What you want is more for less. Regardless of your salary, never forget that this concept is one you must actively practice by being sharp about what is going on around you.

  For example, let's say that your sister's birthday is coming up. At first, you consider buying her an inexpensive present at a discount store. But on second thought, you pick up a newspaper to search for sales. You discover a "75 percent off" sale at an upscale store in the mall. You visit the store and buy a nice purse marked down from $40 to $10. Thinking ahead has helped you get a super gift, and your budget is still intact.

- **Do you think long term about large purchases?** For instance, let's say that you are newly married. You need new dining room furniture. You're on a tight budget, so you have got to weigh your options carefully. Instead of plunking down money for a cheaper set at the rent-to-own place, you head for a furniture consignment store. You wrangle a super deal on a beautiful oak table and four chairs, which will last a lifetime.

- **Do you know the cumulative value of small amounts of money?** By being careful, let's say that you manage to save $25 per month on your electric bill. Ditto for your groceries. This $50 per month will go into a mutual fund with an 8 percent annual return, compounded monthly. In five years, you'll have over $3,700. You could—among other choices—take a cruise, make a down payment on a house under certain mortgage programs, or start a small business on the side.

  It doesn't matter if you make $20,000 or $200,000 per year, the principles of good money management are the same. You want to cover your real needs, find value, and spend without having too much anxiety about your purchases. In addition, you want to make sure you aren't wasting money or unnecessarily giving it away to your insurance agent, your auto mechanic, or your utility company.

This means that you need to pay attention. For example, monitor where your money goes by writing down everything you spend for three months. Or, routinely begin to compare prices on groceries at different stores to get the most out of every dollar. Pennies saved here and there do add up.

Having major money problems can be deeply frustrating. But the faster you examine your trouble spots, the quicker you can do something about your dilemma. For instance, why not take a look at problems that keep occurring repeatedly. Second, figure out some way to *break the cycle.*

Even if you have an outright financial crisis on your hands, you probably can figure out how to turn it around if you explore your options fully. Try to be objective, and pretend that you are gathering this information for someone else. This helps you stay more coolheaded and logical.

Usually, one small thing is not going to change a crisis. But a *series* of good changes can help turn the tide. These changes don't have to be major ones. They should be very realistic and relatively simple to implement.

> One paramedic we'll call Buddy, says, "I keep charging things on my credit cards. I can't seem to stop. I'm not wasteful and I'm not irresponsible. I truly need more income. After clearing just $1,700 per month, I don't have a lot left because $500 in child support comes out of that.
>
> "I live in a big city where decent housing doesn't come cheap," he continues. "So yes, I'm really strapped for cash."

His answer to stretching his paycheck could be to cut expenses, do without certain things, work a part-time job, or continue to live on credit until that backfires.

If a true lack of income *is* your problem, don't wait for your budget to blow up. For instance, get a roommate to share expenses if you are single. Move closer to work if you are spending lots of money on commuting. Or, if you don't want to work a second job in EMS or fire services, find a part-time job unrelated to emergency work that will help you to develop additional skills—perhaps computer skills or mechanical skills.

If lack of income is your central money problem, you cannot fix it by denial. You cannot fix it by living on credit. Most assuredly, that won't last for long.

> Let's take a look at the creative approach of two EMTs, Craig and Tommy, who wanted to cut their expenses by several hundred dollars a month. Impossible? Not for them. "Tommy and I both come from poor families," says Craig. "We'd lived as neighbors in government housing while growing up. When we both found jobs, we shared a common goal. That goal was to each buy a house for our future families. One night over cards Tommy said to me, 'I've got an idea about how we could build a nest egg for ourselves. I want you to hear my plan.' "
>
> Tommy interjects, "I figured out that we could save a lot of money by landing ourselves free housing—and I don't mean the government kind. We became property caretakers for a couple who were going to South America for two years. They were missionaries in our church. I'd overheard them say they wanted people in their home they could trust. When we called them, they were delighted. They felt they could trust two emergency responders to follow through on any agreements."
>
> He continues, "They didn't pay us anything, but we lived rent free, paying only the utility bill. I saved $350 each month for two years, and so did Craig. We

made down payments on small houses at the end of that time. Our houses aren't mansions by anyone's standards. But we're proud of them. You can figure out a lot of ways to cut your expenses if you really need to. First, you have to have a goal that's worth the sacrifice. And a goal should be big enough to drive you. The goal has to say to you, 'Keep going, because you don't want to go back. Go forward.'"

Here's are two techniques to think about for living well on less:

- **Develop good taste.** You can do this by educating yourself about what constitutes good taste. This education costs nothing whatsoever. You can acquire it by doing what some people call "window shopping" or "shopping without money."

  Browse in nice furniture stores and clothing stores. Study magazines while waiting in the doctor's office to get a feel for style on everything. Why? Because you want to *duplicate* good style as closely as possible in less expensive stores.

  For example, you can put together a very classic outfit of gray slacks, a striped shirt, and a navy overcoat from a consignment store for $50. Your friends won't know that you didn't pay $200 for your ensemble, *if you don't tell them.*

  Some antiques stores are great places to buy old glassware or odd pieces of china for $8 or $10. Your friends will be happy to receive well-designed pieces as gifts. Or, use these items to decorate your own home. Flea markets are good places to find old silver pieces or beautiful lamps for affordable prices, too.

- **Come up with nice alternatives when money is tight. Find a way to enjoy some of the finer things in life by using creativity.**

  "When I was in paramedic training 30 years ago, my wife and I were really scrimping," says Bobby, a responder who now owns two rental houses outright. *"One winter we wanted to visit the ski slopes. Neither of us could ski, which would have been expensive, but we wanted to be in the ski crowd.*

  "We drove to the mountains and spent the afternoon by a big fire in the ski lodge. It was fun watching others come down the slopes through a giant window. We ordered two bowls of chili and lots of hot chocolate. That day was one of the best times we've ever had. I think it cost us a total of twenty dollars."

Making money grow

Educate yourself about building assets and net worth. Your net worth is what you *own* minus what you *owe*. If your home, car, and furniture are worth $100,000, and you owe $70,000 against them, your net worth is $30,000. By acquiring things of value, *which do not readily go down in price,* you are building a good financial base for yourself and your family.

By staying out of debt, you are *protecting* the value of what you have acquired. Your house is an asset. So is your car. But your car, unless it's a classic or an antique, is worth less every day.

Real estate is a more solid investment because it should constantly appreciate, or rise, in value. There will be periods of time—due to high interest rates in your area or a bad economy—when real estate doesn't appreciate. But over the years, it should appreciate at the rate of roughly 3 percent each year.

In some cases, buying undeveloped land can be a good investment. If the taxes each year don't exceed the amount the land increases in value, you are probably going to realize a profit some day. However, there may be years that vacant land might not appreciate in value at all. It is a judgment call for you on whether to purchase raw land. Many people have done so—later realizing a huge profit when a factory or shopping mall wanted the acreage, or a housing developer wanted to put in a subdivision.

However, never buy acreage—or even a vacant lot—without doing tons of research in your community on market trends. Every area in the country is different. Every locale has different industries, businesses, and economic opportunities that govern the outcome of land sales. Make choices in buying housing or land *very care-*

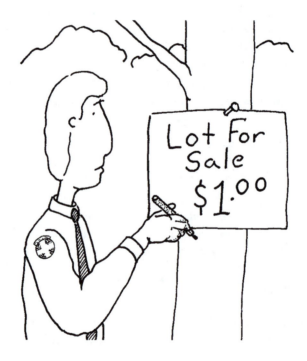

fully. But don't be afraid to take some risks—or you will never improve your financial situation.

> *Chuck, a paramedic from Arizona, was debating on buying a house or a double-wide mobile home a couple of years ago. "I'd inherited a vacant lot worth about $15,000," says Chuck. "An old buddy from high school was selling mobile homes, and he was pressuring me to put a mobile home on the lot. The mobile home unit would have cost around $50,000, not counting the foundation and underpinning. That seemed like too much.*
>
> *"Instead, I sold the lot for $15,000 and paid this money down on a $65,000 house," he explains. "The house needs some cosmetic work, but it's in a good neighborhood. Other houses around me are selling for $80,000. In a few years, I believe my house will be worth $100,000. That mobile home will probably be worth less than half that."*

Chuck is probably very wise in making the decision he did. Houses typically do appreciate in value about 3 percent per year. Investing in a traditional home has worked well for most people because making payments on a house is a "forced investment." Most people don't have the discipline to save and invest money over the years that would equal the equity they would have in a house.

Money moves need to be as carefully planned as moving pieces on a chessboard. Every move *does* count. Keep in mind that you will make two kinds of money in life: money that you earn from your job and money that *your investments earn.* You will also *lose* money in at least two ways: money you waste through bad purchases or poor judgment, and money *you failed to make* because you did not buy good assets.

Planning is taking control

Working at managing your resources must be a continual effort. It's hard to steer your finances in the right direction without this persistence. Planning on paper is always wise because you can keep track of your progress and enter notes for improvements or changes you would like to try.

As in time management, it helps to have a large notebook where all your financial planning ideas can be kept in one place. Having scraps of paper and ideas in different places will only create confusion.

Budgeting can be worked on more easily if you manage to get an entire mental picture on *one page.* For example, in a financial planning notebook, list all of your income and debts on one page. Also, track your monthly utility bills on one page. Or, enter on a single page the amount you're spending for groceries every month. This kind of tracking will help you to see if your expenses there are getting out of control.

If they are, you can plan to work at trimming your utility bill. Or, you might want to stop buying too many expensive convenience foods at the grocery store.

Ask yourself, "What *small but consistent things* could I do, or have my family do, to ensure we'll have some money to save?" Don't increase your stress levels by making plans that are overly optimistic. Don't neglect your situation by believing there's nothing you can do. If you search hard enough, you can find ways to manage well on a small salary.

You can buy a house, save money, travel, and take care of your family if you make a plan to find and manage resources. For example, if you want to buy a home like Craig and Tommy above both managed to do, you could possibly do property caretaking to save money. Or, if you're an EMT who wants to become a paramedic, there may be hospitals in your area that will help finance your education.

If you would like to save on everyday items, there are excellent Web sites to visit on the Internet to guide you on finding bargains. There are sites for purchasing almost any item you can name—from cars to pets—on the Internet. If you're not computer literate, find a friend who is and ask him or her to help you locate what you need.

Debt concept

Many young responders who are new to the world of managing finances often ask, "Is it bad to be in debt?" Those who have sought credit counseling, especially, feel confused about how to use debt as a tool. The answer to the question concerning debt is: Debt, by itself, is not a destructive thing. Mismanaged debt or too much debt is.

Debt, carefully worked into your budget, can even help you build wealth. For example, at some point in your life, buying a rental house in addition to your present home can be a wise move for your retirement years. Or, buying a profitable business can be done through acquiring debt.

Everyone—even those individuals with very small salaries—should learn to handle small amounts of debt. Debt helps you establish a good credit rating, which is an invaluable asset. A good credit rating can help you buy a house, a car, or acquire an educational loan.

> *"Always keep your credit good with your plumber, your auto mechanic, and your banker," laughs Ed, a young firefighter from Illinois. "I remember when I was newly married and living in a tiny cold house one winter. The pipes burst. The bill was high because the plumber had to come out on Sunday. Plus, it took him hours to maneuver himself in and out of the tight crawl space to fix the broken pipes.*
>
> *"When he handed me the bill, I nearly fainted," Ed continues. "It was $170. I had no cash. My checking account had $30 in it. I could see myself facing a cop*

before the day was over. I stammered something like, 'Uh . . . could I make this in payments?' "

"The plumber said, 'Well, I don't usually do business that way. But I'll make an exception in your case. My brother knows you. He worked on your car recently. He told me before I left home that you were good for the money.' "

Reminder

Unless you're rich, you are not going to live very comfortably without planned, well-managed debt. Your credit rating is an incredibly valuable tool. If your credit rating is flawed, work diligently for the next 12 to 18 months to get your payments made on time. Overdue notations will move off of your credit rating eventually. Most creditors look at the past year when deciding to lend money.

So what if you are head over heels in debt now? Let's say that your many credit cards are up to their limit. Your total credit debt is crushing you. If you can get a home equity loan to clean up those debts, that's probably your best alternative. Just remember to break the cycle that got you overloaded to begin with—impulse spending, carrying too many credit cards, or using credit as a false income.

If you can't get a home equity loan, visit your Consumer Credit Counseling Service, a nonprofit organization. Its advice is absolutely free, and this agency will help you look at new options. It may even be able to assist you in getting some of your monthly payments reduced without harming your credit. Never be embarrassed about having money problems, but do take responsibility for getting free counseling, even if you must drive to a neighboring town to meet with an adviser.

Financial stress is so hard for anyone that it can almost be worse than a physical illness. Money worries will keep you constantly under stress. By learning new skills, taking charge of your spending, and quickly seeking advice or help if you need it, you can turn your finances into a manageable part of your life.

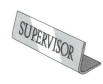

If you are an EMS supervisor, it can also be tempting to ignore departmental budget problems when you're pressed for time. "It's easy to put off doing things, such as writing letters to organizations who can help you gain donations," says Frank, an EMS director over a small county. "When I first began my career, I was trained by an old tightwad in my town to be a money-conscious manager. At the time, I thought this man was a worrywart and a royal pain. I got so mad because he'd constantly nag me to watch the bottom line. I'm now thankful I paid attention.

"Young managers today must keep that ink in the black," he continues. "Too many services get into trouble because they wait too long to cry 'wolf.' "

He continues, "There are government programs for recovering funds your department spends in a disaster. There are cost recovery fees for hazardous materials incidents to keep track of. Even the United Way or Community Chest in your area can't help you unless you stay on top of those things. Money is out there, but you have to go after it. Managers must be aggressive about looking for resources."

Whether you are just beginning your career as a supervisor or you are further along, it can be easy to forget how important it is to locate resources. Successful people must utilize both conventional and unconventional resources to help themselves. Remember that resources can be those *people* in social or business circles who can help you. Or, organizations, such as large companies or schools that supply funding to you or your department, can be labeled as resources.

Another resource is your own individual creativity, because everything that happens in the career world or your personal life materializes from a spark of ingenuity in the human brain. It always helps to be creative in designing exactly what you want for yourself or your department. Then be very proactive in trying to access resources to support those plans.

For example, if your department needs more vehicles for working events that attract large crowds, don't forget that surplus equipment can be purchased at military bases. Also, old buses and other vehicles can be converted into EMS vehicles or rolling "offices." Sharing equipment with other nearby departments can work in some instances to save money. A few EMS departments have even helped in movie productions to raise cash for certain projects.

A helpful resource

One helpful publication, which is a collective reference of ideas compiled by departments from every state, offers a multitude of strategies for raising capital and temporary cash for your EMS or fire division. Bound in three-ring notebook form, it is available from the U.S. Fire Administration. This material, titled *A Guide to Funding Alternatives for Fire and Emergency Medical Services Departments,* can be obtained by writing to Funding Alternatives Project Officer, U.S. Fire Administration, 16825 S. Seton Avenue, Emmitsburg, Maryland 21727.

REVIEW ACTIVITIES

1. Why is it important to appear well-organized at work?
2. List three ways you could manage your time better.

3. Name one area of your financial picture that you would like to improve. Whom could you contact for help or advice with your problem?

4. Name two ways you could save a total of $30 per month. Can you think of additional ways to save even more?

5. Do you have enough organizational tools in your work environment? If not, does this add to your stress levels?

6. List three areas of your home life that could benefit from implementing better planning. Are these areas related to time management, money management, or both?

7. Let's say that you want to save one hour per week on running errands. How could you devise a plan for managing your stops more efficiently? How could you enlist your family's participation?

8. If you want to buy a house soon, how could you organize a plan to make that a reality? What people in your area could you contact to learn more about how to make such a plan?

9. What is the definition of net worth? What are two ways you could increase your net worth over the next 10 years?

FOR SUPERVISORS

1. Notice which of your scheduling problems keeps recurring. Keep track of what isn't working when it comes to staying ahead of the clock. Then figure out a way to break the cycle. For example, if all of your ambulances are in need of tune-ups at the same time, why not have them serviced on Wednesdays and Thursdays? (Depending on the number of vehicles you have, you might give attention to two or three vehicles on these days every other week. That way, they could all be serviced on a regular basis.)

2. Let's say that you want to advance to a higher position in the next three years. Make a plan for organizing goals that could help you achieve this. Break each of those goals down into manageable parts. Assign a deadline to each step of every individual goal.

CLASS PROJECTS

1. Have all class members list one or two ways each one feels disorganized. Then ask everyone to exchange this list with a fellow classmate. Have students offer tips to assist each other in becoming better organized.

2. Discuss the importance of spending money wisely. For example, how can an individual benefit by comparison shopping for clothes, food, and cars?

3. Have the class discuss the importance of living within one's means.

CHAPTER EIGHT

ASSESSING YOUR CAREER STRESS

Has reporting for work become a real grind? You may not be a candidate for full-scale burnout, but you don't feel the enthusiasm you once did for your job. Sometimes you tell yourself, "I'm lucky to have this job." The next minute you groan, "I feel trapped."

Getting into a job rut will eventually happen to almost anyone in any profession. That boxed-in feeling of "the job owns me" or "I'm just spinning my wheels" is one of the worst feelings any worker can have. But by thoroughly assessing your situation, you can find control measures to lower your stress. If you're really burning out on the job, it will probably take *less energy* to plow out of a job rut than to stay stuck.

Initially, it will take effort and careful planning to change something, but the payoffs will be well worth it. You'll end up with more energy, not to mention greater self-esteem, when you get to a better place in your career. You don't necessarily have to change jobs. You don't necessarily have to do anything major. When you take an honest look at what's going on, you can outline changes that can make a difference in how you feel.

Here are just a few reasons you can feel
job dissatisfaction:

- Being around negative people
- Having unfulfilled dreams
- Feeling that you're on the wrong career track
- Fearing that you will lose your job for any number of reasons
- Comparing yourself to someone who's more successful

"It's easy to feel bad about your job when you compare yourself to those who are more successful," says Bryan, who recently retired from the military. He now works in an EMS management position in the Great Lakes region. "When I got out of high school in 1971, I used to see this classmate of mine driving a brand-new red Corvette. He told me he was building houses with his uncle. He said he was clearing 1500 dollars a week. That was a fortune back then. I was clearing 100 dollars a week as a gopher in a medical clinic. I remember thinking, 'How can I get into building houses?' "

"One Sunday morning, I fixed the last two eggs I had. I slapped the morning paper down beside my plate. As I nibbled my breakfast, my mind kept going back to my rich friend. I kept thinking I should ask him more about his job—until I flipped the paper over. His picture was glaring back at me. He had been arrested for dealing drugs. Since then," laughs Bryan, "I've trusted my own career choices."

Like Bryan, we can all get into the mode of comparing ourselves to others. Although it's good to observe what others are doing, it never is wise to believe we would fit into a certain niche just because someone else does. It's very important to be able to do work you enjoy, even if the pay isn't astronomical.

It also is helpful to be aware of the type of people you want to work with. You will absorb many of the *feelings and beliefs* of those in your company. Being around negative coworkers can greatly contribute to your feeling depressed about your job. Associating with positive people can have the opposite effect. A positive person's attitude can energize you in a way that nothing else can.

"I was on the verge of quitting EMS last year," explains Ron, a veteran of 25 years. "I was working with two responders who are both very nice people. But both of these men had gone through divorce. Their bad luck was impacting me. Their ex-wives were constantly calling our station to cry and carry on. One of these women came down to the station one night with her new boyfriend. She wanted to flaunt her new love to her ex. The quarrel that ensued was so bad, I ended up having to help bodily throw this boyfriend out of the station."

He continues, "Well, I knew I needed a change. I asked my boss to transfer me to a different station a few miles east. This new station looks out on a beautiful view of the mountains. There's always something fun going on here. The employees are building furniture for the station, and I'm helping them. I'm having a ball learning to make this great Indian-looking 'twig' furniture.

"I took a chance in switching stations, because I didn't really know what the new environment would be like. I just wanted out of the old place. But, the people I work with now are cheerful about everything. When I go home, I can't wait to get back here."

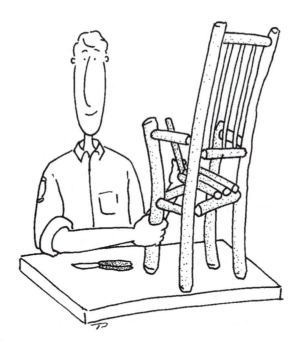

As in Ron's situation, sometimes a single change will add up significantly in lowering stress. Or, a series of small changes might do the trick. For example, you might need to swap certain tasks with someone else. Maybe you're tired of tracking supplies and helping with quality assurance. You would rather be on the fund-raising committee. Or, you want your name in the pot to work an upcoming political rally. In addition, you might want to find part-time work one day a week in a hospital ICU or ER to develop new skills. On top of this, you might decide to start researching jobs in the health-care professions, so that you can begin planning a different career track to be on four years from now.

Consider these suggestions if you feel trapped in your job:

- **When you're against a brick wall, find a mentor.** If you're fresh out of ideas, admit it. All of us will reach a point where we cannot see beyond our present situation. If you're stuck in a very big way, you will get nowhere by asking yourself the same questions over and over. A mentor may have answers and options you never would think of on your own. If possible, get two or three career mentors.
- **Select a mentor *who has nothing to gain or lose by helping you.*** You probably should not make your immediate supervisor a mentor. His or her helping you to make significant career changes or advance to a dif-

ferent position might be a "conflict of interest." Your supervisor's job is to help you do your present job well. Go outside of your department, if possible, to find mentors.

- **Do ask advice from your supervisor on how to make small changes.** It's okay to say to him or her, "I need something to add a little pizzazz to my job." He or she can give you something new to do, while redirecting some of your tasks to someone else.

- **Look at the broadest career picture you possibly can.** You need to research your choices fully and take responsibility for doing that. Attend EMS conferences and read EMS magazines. Buy or borrow good books on career planning in the health-care field. Get your name on mailing lists to obtain newsletters from public safety organizations and hospitals. Figure out *all* of the possibilities for employment that are related to where your interests lie.

Making the decision to continue working as a street medic or to leave the street action for work in management or another field should not cause you undue stress. That's not to say that you won't have to do some intense *soul searching*. You might even have moments of anguish about making a change. But your decisions should be easier, if you do your homework. Talk with your mentors to evaluate your choices properly.

If you understand the price you'll have to pay for change, you can make the decision to pay that price more wholeheartedly. For instance, your schedule may have to change significantly in order to work somewhere else. You may have to come in on your days off to learn a new role. Or, you might have to commit to obtaining more formal education if you want to hit the next rung of the career ladder.

If you stay in your present job, you want to stay for the *right reasons*. If you leave, you want to leave for the right reasons—to go to a position where you will feel better about yourself and more in harmony with your deepest desires. You will feel less stress over the long haul when you make educated choices that are right for you.

IT'S NEVER TOO LATE

"I was very burned out by the time I retired," says Victor, a paramedic who worked one full-time and one part-time job for many years. "I felt like I'd be one of those people who'd die soon after retirement. Anyway, I was depressed, and that's an understatement. To tell the truth, I started drinking heavily because my wife was ill at the time. I was really under a lot of strain financially. I felt angry that I'd spent my life just earning a buck.

"Of course, we all have to get paid. But I was one of these people with unfulfilled dreams burning within me. It hurt me terribly to just forget them, because it's

like losing a part of yourself. I'd sit in my den and smoke three packs of cigarettes a day just reflecting on why I burned out on the job. I kept looking back at the expectations I'd had at a much younger age."

He continues, "What I'd envisioned as a young medic was that I could make a difference in the future of EMS. I'm mechanically inclined, and I'd wanted to design new equipment—perhaps making a real difference in saving lives or being remembered for something I'd invented. That sounds egotistical, I know. But I had started in EMS with these large ambitions. No one I ever worked with encouraged me at all. In fact, a lot of them brushed me off when I'd talk about inventing something.

"Well, two years after I retired, I learned about an interesting bunch of people. A group of responders and health-care professionals in a neighboring county were designing and marketing new EMS and hospital equipment. These people were getting a lot of recognition in EMS journals and in the local news. On a whim, I called one of them to ask if I could meet with them. I blurted out that I wanted to help them free of charge. I thought they might think I was silly for acting this way, but they didn't. They were very supportive. I jumped in and become part of their team.

"I'm now earning a little bit of money, and I expect to earn more. We have an attorney who is helping us with the legal and financial parts of our business. I just designed a new piece of equipment for our local hospital, and they gave me a bonus check for $15,000. As long as you're reasonably healthy, it's never too late to do some exciting things."

If you're feeling stuck and unmotivated, you need to examine your part in how you got into this mode. After all, each of us can contribute to our stressful state in the workplace by failing to be proactive for change. It can be easier to become passive and simply let things happen to us.

Here are several ideas for reflecting on why your stress levels may be too high:

- **Work can get boring if you're not making a unique contribution.** By offering something special of yourself—a talent for coordinating committees or for helping to plan educational seminars—you'll feel more stimulated. If you're a creative person, too much routine work will dampen your spirits.

- **Expecting too much from a single job will practically guarantee that you will feel lots of stress.** *No job* is so fulfilling that it will meet all of your emotional needs. By opening yourself up to exploring new hobbies, mastering new skills in the workplace, and meeting new people, you will find more balance.

- **If you're not having pleasant experiences outside of work, your job probably won't feel as rewarding.** Every week, try to monitor your overall experiences to ensure that something nice is taking place in your life.

When life is hectic, it becomes harder to work pleasant experiences into your schedule. However, even a two-hour walk through a park once a week can help. If you can manage something as uplifting as canoeing down a lazy river, you're probably going to *sail* through some of your workdays.

"I was so sick of my job I prayed for aliens to abduct me," laughs Fran, a paramedic from Florida. "I was in full-scale burnout last year. I had no enthusiasm for hearing about career goals or career anything.

"My sister knew how badly I felt, so she starting asking me a few questions over the phone one night. She asked me if I really hated my job—or had I just been neglecting myself. She asked if I was eating right and exercising. Well, I wasn't. I thought about this the rest of the evening.

"My diet—soft drinks, potato chips, too many white bread sandwiches—was pitiful. My exercise program didn't exist. I saw what my sister was trying to tell me. You're not going to love your job if you don't feel well.

"I started eating fruits and vegetables and running three days a week. I got a new haircut. I bought some new clothes. After a month of taking better care of myself, I didn't feel so burned out about the job. I still don't love the job I'm in, but I feel okay about it. I feel more in control of everything because I'm taking better care of me."

If you are in full-scale burnout at any point in your career, reflect on these strategies for getting off overload:

- **You must back away from burnout in stages.** You didn't get to this point overnight, and you won't end it overnight. It will take lots of small changes, *which are well integrated into your normal routine,* before you will feel a lot better. Coping with true job burnout is seldom a one-step process.
- **Finding control in *several* areas of your life will help to ease job burnout.** Just fixing things at work won't necessarily help you feel harmonious. Job burnout usually leads to a depressed state that affects *all areas* of life. Try to make at least two or three small, positive changes in several areas—in your work situation, your personal relationships, your self-care program—in order to move slowly in the right direction.
- **Don't overwhelm yourself with too many goals at once.** When you feel desperate about your stress levels, you can vow to change 10 things at

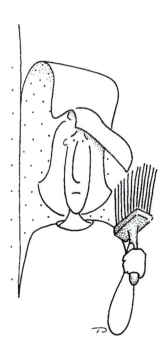

once, and you'll probably fail. Try two or three and make them stick. Then try more.

Also, when you're in a very intense state of job burnout, it can be tempting to throw yourself into demanding goals elsewhere. At home, for example, you might try to remodel five rooms all at once. Or, on impulse, you may find yourself volunteering to help on five committees at your child's school.

Why would you overload yourself this way? Because focusing on your *new stress* helps you to deny your job stress. You can push it aside and tell yourself you'll deal with it in the future. But it's better to evaluate your job pressures and plan a few productive changes. Your job burnout will start to subside when you feel a slightly new *enthusiasm* for work.

How gung-ho are you?

"I believe that work is a lot like Christmas shopping," says Kate, a first responder. "If you go at it halfheartedly, you can't stand it. I remember one Christmas, I heard somebody say, 'Don't moan and groan. Either throw yourself into Christmas shopping with the enthusiasm of a child—or don't do it at all.' Well, I tried it. It worked. That was the first Christmas I'd enjoyed in years. I started applying this theory to cooking for my family, fixing up my house, and dealing with my patients. When I jump in with enthusiasm, everything becomes a whole lot easier."

Tackling a job with vigor is great, if you can do it. But when a job becomes monotonous, it can also help to enlarge your perception of *who you are.* You can gain a new sense of self by figuring out ways to grow and develop. Target something new to do. Then maybe you'll feel some of your old enthusiasm returning.

For example, a job can feel stifling if you don't feel challenged intellectually by it. Every person will mentally outgrow parts of his or her job. Each of us, from time to time, needs new directions, new challenges, and a fresh way to focus personal talents and skills.

Like Ken Kerr, a paramedic from the Knoxville, Tennessee, area, you might combine your love of photography with EMS. Ken was selected by a professional journal to photograph EMS activities at the 1996 Olympics in Atlanta. Ken has furnished many cover shots for magazines such as *Journal of Emergency Medical Services (JEMS)* and the former *Emergency* magazine.

Or, like Alan Azzara, you might figure out a way to combine your writing skills with EMS. Alan left the big-city life as a New York attorney to run an ambulance business in Freeport, Maine. He has written articles on EMS law and a book on the legal issues of EMS. In addition, he's written a pharmacology reference guide for responders by teaming up with a physician who agreed to co-author the book.

In your own situation, could you pair up with another professional in EMS or in a related field to teach a special course—maybe getting paid a nice fee for doing so? Or, could you contribute livesaving tips or fire safety tips to a business newsletter or an insurance company leaflet? Could you organize a collection of police, fire, and EMS tools for a city event—or perhaps be instrumental in starting a museum of such tools and equipment?

If you are in a job rut, or trapped in full-blown burnout, think of this dilemma as a catalyst for change. After all, massive frustration is a very strong sign that something hasn't been working for some time. You don't necessarily have to switch jobs, get promoted, or take on profound challenges. You can work for change right where you are.

Here are three ways to work at developing yourself in your present situation, if your job is unrewarding:

- **Expand your present job by focusing on new projects—with your supervisor's permission, of course.** Look for anything to give you a new direction, even if the project is a very simple one. Your goal is not to become thrilled by your new work. Your goal is to feel that you have the *power to create change* in your work setting.

- **Augment your present job with a part-time job that is significantly different from what you have been doing.** There is nothing like diversity to pull you out of a depressed state. Focusing too much on EMS will destroy the beauty of the job. Eating, sleeping, and dreaming about running calls or managing a response unit will backfire after a time. If you go into overkill about *anything,* you will probably tire of it.

- **Do some volunteer work in your professional community.** Find your way into a hospital setting, a police precinct, or someplace where you will be exposed to learning new skills. If your present job isn't that exciting, you should expose yourself to various other work arenas. Work hard to learn new skills that you can add to your résumé. The more skills you have, the more marketable you will be if you want to change jobs.

Working in the fire services or emergency response will open lots of doors for you. Everyone from your local movie theater owner to the town's best restaurateur might claim friendship with you. There is nothing wrong with using your clout to enter new territory.

These tips can get you moving:

- **Be an opportunist.** Take advantage of what comes up. If you enjoy politics, go to city council meetings. Chat with city officials and learn what drives the political machine of your area. Serve on a committee in your community to learn leadership skills.

    Want to try your hand at journalism? Crank out a column on safety for your local newspaper. Ask a local high school English teacher to edit it for you. Does business appeal to you? Plan a fund-raiser for your fire station. You could have an auction with items donated by local businesses. Why not try serving as auctioneer?

- **Create a group effort.** Dig out of a job rut by helping to bring small successes to your division. Organize a team of people to accomplish something interesting. For example, one group of paramedics in Tennessee had fun fixing a problem that came up every year: How could they transport the sick and injured out of the crowds during their town's annual Springfest? The medics got busy converting used golf carts bought at a state park into mobile EMS units. From there, they converted used buses, cars, and station wagons into various EMS vehicles that each served a need.

- **Take some pressure off the boss.** Why not expand your job by figuring out a way to create win–win situations for yourself and your supervisor. "My supervisor dreads speaking in public," says one paramedic. "So I volunteer to give talks for schools and civic clubs. My motive? I plan to be a sales rep for a pharmaceutical company in the future. Anytime I speak, I'm polishing my public relations skills."

> Any choices you make about supplementary employment should meet some of your *deeper psychological needs* that your present job cannot. Work-related stress won't necessarily put you into a job rut. However, *not getting your emotional needs met* will.

Volunteering opens doors

"Well," you might say, "all these ideas about broadening your horizons wouldn't help me. I'm stuck in a low-paying job in a rural fire station. The opportunities here are limited."

In this case, your best bet might be to do volunteer work with other agencies in your area. Volunteering can often be a great educational ticket when you don't necessarily want to go back into a formal classroom.

Even if you must drive 30 miles to a hospital, university, or police department, it can be worth the effort. You can gain computer skills, social skills, business training, and knowledge of management by donating your talents.

When you do volunteer, here's how to invest your efforts for real payoffs:

- **Run with the movers and shakers.** Try to associate with good role models. Notice how self-assured people handle stressful phone calls, difficult coworkers, and heavy workloads. Their skills will rub off on you.
- **Keep your ear to the ground.** Every day, pay close attention to what is going on around you. Pick up on any opportunities to work with professionals who might help you do more.
- **Document your new skills.** Keep a written journal of those skills you are adding to your knowledge bank. If you are involved in assessing patient needs in some way or helping to do telephone triage work, write these skills down so that you can add them to your résumé.

Try to do something uplifting

"I was forcing myself to get out of bed every day," says Cliff, an EMT who considered quitting many times. "I was burning out, in part, because our station felt like a center for social problems. We had this enormous problem with needy people and elderly people in our community calling us because they were lonely or upset. It was a real abuse of the system.

"My sister-in-law, who is a social worker, challenged me to help her create a program for the elderly. She said, 'We'll solicit volunteers to check in on these people by phone twice a day.' She had read up on how this was being done in other parts of the country. At first, I resented her invitation to participate. Exhausted, burned out people don't like hearing the words 'more work.' But once I got involved, I felt better. I'm learning a lot of skills in working with older people. There are many job opportunities in working with the elderly, and I'm considering one or two options in that direction for the future."

Recipe for self-defeat

You will be guaranteed to stay locked in career stress of any kind if you assume a passive role. Not making a choice *is* a real decision. By doing nothing, you're agreeing that you will accept the status quo.

In order to become an advocate for your own career, you will need to reverse self-defeating behaviors. In Chapter 1, we talked about some of those. As a quick refresher, let's review them again:

- Believe you're nobody special. Just keep thinking there's nothing really unique about you. Make average goals and lead an average life. Never try to stand out.

- Always please the crowd. Never ask yourself, "What do I need from life and from work?" If the boss is happy, your spouse is happy, and your kids are happy, this means that you're okay.

- Limit your education to a classroom. Never pick up a book, read a piece of literature, or learn anything beyond what's required.

- Cling to your comfort zone. Never put any extra pressure on yourself. Do the absolute minimum you can to get by.

- Refuse to conquer your fears. Don't try to get over your fear of public speaking. Let opportunities to teach pass you by. Feel intimidated by computers? Stay away from computer classes. Let somebody else study software programs that might help your department.

GO FOR THE GOLD

Whenever you make a decision to grab for the brass ring—or perhaps the gold one—you are going to have to sacrifice something. You'll have to spend time, money, or energy in the short term to gain what you want. Nothing happens without giving up something. You have to *give* in order to receive the rewards you want. Larger goals are never easy to attain. But neither is staying stuck. If you strive for bigger goals, however, you will wind up with more overall *life satisfaction*.

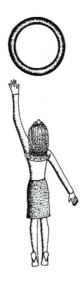

Keep in mind as you assess your career situation that plenty of EMTs are happy in their roles for 35 years. If you are one of them, celebrate the fact that you're not stressed about leaving that role. Changing from a role you enjoy probably *will not* lower your stress. In fact, it may increase it significantly. If you have no desire to be a supervisor or to be in management, you can spend your energy in other ways.

Many EMS personnel in management positions were happier *before* they got promoted. If you're one of them, you might eventually want to go back to running calls. Asking to be demoted or rerouted can be tricky because of politics or your financial considerations. But if you *intensely dislike your job,* don't hesitate to consider doing your old one.

Remember that the *tasks* you do comprise your job—not your job description. Always identify the day-to-day agenda that most appeals to you. If you enjoy a hectic schedule of running continual calls, that's great. But if that schedule loses its appeal after a while, you would be wise to acknowledge that you need a change. Too many people have quit EMS impulsively because they didn't know how to make a change. Taking time to think and plan is the key to maintaining job satisfaction—wherever you want to be on the career ladder.

Doing a job assessment

You don't want to create *more stress* for yourself by repeatedly saying, "I'm not happy with my job." But if this is the case, go ahead and acknowledge the reality of your situation. Think of your honesty as your wake-up call to assess your career fully. Even if you tremendously *enjoy* what you're doing, it still is good to assess your job and your long-term career track periodically. No one should let a lot of time go by without spending some time on career planning.

Whatever you want to do, you can attain the opportunities with enough planning. You might not reach all of your goals perfectly. Few people do. But you can achieve enough of your goals to find balance and feel better about yourself.

EMS is a field that interfaces with many other professions, so you probably have *more choices* than the average American worker to find employment when your present job, for some reason, might be ending. Fears concerning company downsizing or managed care and how those dollars will be distributed to EMS might not be idle fears. All sorts of changes will be taking place in the financial picture of EMS and related professions for years to come. But knowing how to define your skills and sell them to an employer will help you curb anxiety. Even a little more self-confidence makes it easier to open a new door.

> *"I panicked seven years ago, because I lost my job," says Paige, a responder whose parents both work in EMS. "A new company had acquired our ambulance service. The new boss cleaned house. My head was the first to roll. I was worried I'd never find another job in our small county.*
>
> *"I stayed up all night pacing the floor because I didn't know what to do. My dad came over the next morning to set me straight. 'You've got to put together a résumé and document your skills,' he instructed. 'Believe you're going to find a job, because you deserve to. Act like you deserve to. Write your résumé like you deserve to.' I followed his advice, and by the end of the week, I got employed in the Sleep Studies Center of a hospital in a neighboring town. The job only lasted two years, but it paid my bills until I could get back into EMS."*

In order to stay employed, you need to be informed about selling your talents. For example, if you're good at mentoring others, or you can bring demanding projects to completion, put these skills on your résumé. Coaching others well is an impressive skill. Being able to manage large projects requires very unique talents. These talents would include, among others, that you be self-directed, disciplined, and methodical.

Evaluating your job skills and your life skills requires objectivity. A good mentor can help you review your old résumé and work on updating it. He or she can instruct you further on identifying more skills to list on your résumé. If you don't fully evaluate yourself, you can fail to market yourself properly when you must change jobs.

> *"I believe that competition in the workplace is positive in a lot of ways," says Christine, a paramedic who would like to work for an EMS consulting firm someday. "Competition for employment seems scary, but skilled medics are going to find their place in the sun. Of course, you have to be flexible."*
>
> *Christine often talks with administrators at two EMS consulting firms in her area. "I tell them to keep me in mind for any position they have," she explains. "You have to let people know what your career plans are. My son left for college*

last year, and I'm at the point where I can be flexible. My husband has a good job, which he can keep, if either of these two firms decides to hire me.

"I use every spare second to study the future of EMS. I know details about the latest equipment, all of the best manufacturers, budgets for large and small services, and a lot more. You should see the literature I have in my home office. I believe I can make a contribution in the consulting area, so I'll keep pushing until I open some kind of door."

With her enthusiasm, Christine probably will eventually land a job with an EMS consulting firm. An upbeat approach doesn't hurt a thing. When you feel upbeat, your personal energy is higher. You can think more clearly. You also will probably make more exciting goals.

If you need to motivate yourself to change, think about the frame of mind that will help you. Think about these ways to drive yourself in the right direction:

- **Make goals that are believable and achievable *for you.*** By selecting a goal that is tailor-made for your energy levels, your deepest desires, and your true life situation, you will be able to give it your full support. That's not to say that you won't have to make yourself uncomfortable to achieve it. No one can stay in a comfort zone and reach a goal of any size, but it should fit in with an overall balanced plan for your life. You want to be able to carry the goal to completion.

- **Look at your support system.** For example, let's say that you are the single parent of three small children. If your support system for child care is shaky, you will have to get your support in place *before* you make a higher commitment. Too many people in this situation have gotten into school or a demanding job that they wound up having to quit. If they had researched their options fully, they probably would have been able to make their plans work.

  If you are a parent without extended family or good support, research your options for child care thoroughly. Figure out all of the alternatives in your community. Talk to others who have been in a similar situation. However, *don't wait until your plan is flawless* because that seldom happens. But do try to structure a plan that will work.

- **Decide to be highly flexible.** Everything you do will require more effort than you might think. But keep your eye on your goals. When frustration mounts, find a way to be flexible in your thinking or actions. Rigid people usually experience much higher stress levels than those who find a way to steer around the stress.

"Anyone who is successful will have to take some dog bites," laughs Jerry, father of four who now owns an ambulance service with two other investors. "When I was a paramedic, I mortgaged a farm I'd inherited to start this business. In the

Midwest, you don't want to lose the family farm for anything. This new endeavor scared the daylights out of me, but I did it anyway. I was overwhelmed when I tried to pay the bills for the first four years. I had to rob Peter to pay Paul. It was hard, believe me. But now, I'm making a very good living. I haven't lost the farm either.

"I would advise anyone to think more about what they really want to do and less about their fears," Jerry emphasizes. "Your fears are given to you for your protection, so you don't want to discount them totally. But if your fears become your stumbling blocks, you're being ruled by them. If you don't bite off a little more than you can chew, you're not going to get very far."

Reminder

When we plan around our most important goals, we can stand more stress. It is when we are sidetracked by *lesser goals* that we feel used, used up, burned out, and defeated.

Find out how you're misusing your energies. If you're not getting to where you want to go, ask yourself:

- Do I know my top three career goals?
- Do I have time frames in mind for reaching these goals?
- Do I really believe I have the ability to reach these goals?
- What am I doing to work toward them?
- Do I need more educational monies?
- Do I need more people in my support system?

To ensure that you move toward the completion of your goals, spend time reflecting on how you can overcome personal weaknesses, bad habits, or any self-defeating practices. Figure out what you need to do in order to make sure you will reach your goals. For example, do your study habits need improving? Do you need to manage your time better? Do you need to find one or two people who will encourage your efforts?

In Chapter 9, we will discuss how to assess your personal approach to life. After all, you can do a job assessment and make lots of goals—*only to trip yourself up with self-defeating practices*. In order to manage your stress levels or create a new lifestyle, you will be able to succeed when you remove any roadblocks. If those roadblocks lie within you, you have the power to remove them. But you will need to face them head on. A thorough assessment of your approach to challenges, your philosophies about life, and your attitudes toward past experiences can help you overcome any obstacles to success.

In Chapter 10, we will discuss how to create a written plan for both your career and your personal life. Having a true outline of your goals will help you to stay on course. As you implement your plan, keep reminding yourself of why you're making the sacrifices to arrive at where you want to be. Hold yourself accountable. Figure out the steps you need to take. Reach out for help and support when you can't. If one option doesn't work, try another. If one door doesn't open, try another. Never give up on designing the life you want.

REVIEW ACTIVITIES

1. Name three ways that negative coworkers or friends have affected your stress levels recently. Did these experiences impact the productivity of one or more of your workdays? Did these negative individuals cause you to feel negatively about yourself or your job?
2. Why is it important to have a career mentor?
3. Why is it productive to look at a very broad career track, instead of focusing on just one job area in EMS?
4. When your job has become boring, how can volunteering benefit you?
5. Why is it counterproductive to limit your education to a formal classroom?
6. How can having many unique skills increase your marketability to employers?
7. Why is backing away from job burnout seldom a one-step process?
8. Tell why the daily tasks of a particular job will determine much about your job's satisfaction.
9. Name one major goal you might like to achieve. How much sacrifice on your part do you envision this goal would involve? Can you foresee actually paying the price to achieve it?
10. Why should achieving your most important goals, although they may be stressful to accomplish, bring you more overall life satisfaction?

FOR SUPERVISORS

1. You've agreed to mentor a paramedic who wants to make a career change. He or she wants to move into management eventually. What primary questions would you ask this individual? Can you think of ways to help him or her to design goals? Would you share your own successes and failures with this individual? How much would you be willing to share with him or her about the challenges you've faced on your career track?

2. Let's say that you are a supervisor who is facing burnout. Name at least three ways you could enjoy projects outside of EMS. For example, could you organize a hiking club? Could you pursue a hobby with your spouse? Could you try a new sport? Why does it help to put some of your energy into areas outside of work?

CLASS PROJECT

1. Have a member of the class pretend that he or she is very dissatisfied with a specific job in EMS. Have other class members interview this person about the stress. Have the interviewers write questions that would help the unhappy worker assess the true job picture. For example, a student might ask: "If you had a different supervisor, would you be happier in your present role?"

CHAPTER NINE

SELF-ASSESSMENT AND TAKING CONTROL

Plans, goals, and dreams can look great on paper. But if you have self-defeating habits or self-defeating attitudes, you may fail to move ahead. However, when you take full responsibility for improving yourself, you can reach your full potential. You can also decrease your stress levels because you will feel more in control of your destiny.

For example, do you know someone who plays the "blame game"? This person blames the boss, friends, coworkers, or in-laws for his or her troubles. All of us have done this to some degree. After all, other people's actions often do impact us negatively. But if we constantly blame others for our problems, we'll become locked into a victim's role. We'll become victimized instead of being victorious.

Anyone who habitually focuses on the shortcomings of others will thrive on anger. It takes *a ton of energy to feed this anger*. Wasting personal energy this way is a great detriment to reaching goals and managing stress. People who continually blame others can flounder for years, making little progress in their careers or in their personal lives.

"I come from a very dysfunctional family," says Skip, a paramedic–flight nurse. "Years ago, I spent a lot of time blaming my parents for my problems. They didn't really encourage me to try. They never encouraged me to study. When I was 24, I was delivering pizzas for a living. My 12-year-old car was ready for the junkyard.

"One day, I walked into a community college to deliver two pizzas. It was snowing outside. The roads were getting slicker by the minute. I was worried I'd slide off the road on my way back to the restaurant. But in reality, I was worried I was sliding off of a bigger cliff.

"I asked the girl behind the desk, 'Do you have anybody here who could get me going in the right direction? I need to quit this pizza job.'

"She said, 'If you're serious, you've come to the right place.'

"When the snow melted, I went back to talk with an adviser. He signed me up for one class which met two nights a week. I told him, 'My parents didn't encourage me to study. They weren't into education all that much. I don't know if I can do this.'

"The adviser stood up and walked closer to me. He put his hand firmly on my shoulder and said, 'You can't blame your parents anymore. You outgrew them when you walked in this door.'"

Skip has done freelance writing for EMS publications. He serves on three committees for planning EMS conferences in his region. He has won several awards for working with the Parent–Teacher Organization in his city. The only pizza he delivers now is the one he brings home to his wife and two children. Skip says the lesson he's learned over the past few years is this: The most immediate power you have at your disposal is the power to change yourself.

Any kind of self-defeating patterns—engaging in poor habits, looking on the dark side of things, failing to discipline yourself—can keep you from reaching your goals. Spinning your wheels, instead of getting to where you want to go, will create so much cumulative stress that you'll be facing *burnout* before you find your *way out*.

SO HOW ARE YOUR HABITS?

Let's examine your personal habits for a moment. Are you doing anything that could deter progress in your career? Or, are you caught up in negative patterns that create stress in your personal life?

For example, let's hypothesize that you smoke three packs of cigarettes a day. One repercussion from this would be that smoking is costing you several hundred dollars per year. This will affect your finances. In addition, this habit might be keeping you from running or doing a vigorous exercise program. Perhaps you have tried several times to beat your habit by quitting "cold turkey." But after a day or two, you always caved in and smoked twice as much to make up for the days you abstained.

If quitting suddenly hasn't ended your habit, why not make a different plan? Could you gradually switch to light cigarettes and then ultralights? Could you wear a nicotine patch with the goal of switching to lower dosages over time?

The point is, it will take a concerted effort to direct yourself away from self-defeat. Whether you smoke too many cigarettes or try to accommodate too many people during the course of a workday, your overdoing may very well affect the larger picture of your life. Remember that your habits in life will make you or break you.

If you can picture life as a rowboat, try to envision how your habits might be the oars of this craft. It's your habits that propel you in certain directions. It's what you *consistently do right* that will push you in the desired directions. Without the proper habits, you may row around in circles.

If you are off course in your personal habits, or your personal approach to life, you must diligently pursue those methods that will ensure your success. By improving one or two small habits, you will gain more control. If you can reverse several bad habits, you'll probably get the upper hand on a lot of stress.

Think about how much stress you're experiencing right now because you're failing to clear a certain hurdle in your life. Maybe you want a better relationship with your mate or you may want a higher-paying position in your career. Ask yourself, "Are my habits preventing me from having what I want?" For instance, do you criticize your significant other too much? Or, do you constantly rub your boss the wrong way?

If you do need to change, focus on how you can interrupt the cycles that are making you repeatedly do the same wrong things. Monitor your own performance for improving all aspects of your life. For instance, develop the habit of looking for every opportunity to compliment your spouse. Or, start doing everything you can to create good feelings among your coworkers.

Reminder

Don't feel badly if you have tried and failed to break a bad habit. Remember to *keep trying*. You will eventually find a way to succeed. Don't give up until you break through the wall or jump the hurdle that's defeating you.

Let's take a closer look at some bad habits which could increase your stress levels:

- **Do you constantly rehearse your failures?** Individuals who keep dwelling on their mistakes are wasting the only resource they can never replace—time. Although you can beg, borrow, or steal money—or almost any other resource—time is one resource that you can *never retrieve*. Learn quickly from your mistakes and drop them. Move on to more productive pursuits.

- **Are you constantly pushing to keep busy?** In certain instances, keeping busy may actually *prevent* true accomplishment. Just expending energy doesn't mean that you are efficient. Occasionally slow down to evaluate what's going on. Assess whether or not you are getting *results* from your endeavors.

- **Do you often look for the easy way out?** It's okay to cut corners on some of the activities you need to accomplish. But be careful that you do hold yourself accountable for tackling important tasks with precision. If you do things halfway, you will probably wind up having to do a lot of them over. This will intensify stress.

"I remember working with this middle-aged man who always did the absolute minimum he could to get by. We'll call him Speedy," laughs Lisa, a nurse who began her career as an EMT. "We had two ambulances at our tiny substation. One afternoon, the boss asked Speedy to change the oil in one of those vehicles. Well, he drained out the old oil, but he didn't add any back. Knowing him, he was going to ask someone on the next shift to do it.

"We got a call where a patient wound up in full arrest one street away from the station. We hopped in one of the ambulances, and I started to crank her up. But Speedy screamed, 'Wait! There's no oil in this thing!' We had to scramble into the other vehicle and hightail it. I told myself right then, I'd never be one of those people who scrapes by doing the minimum. That's a recipe for disaster."

Working to change self-defeating habits means that you are *working to become your best self.* Self-improvement will help you feel more in control of your life. As you change in positive ways—whether by practicing productive habits or by becoming a better communicator—everyone and everything around you will seem to change for the better.

When you become tired of what isn't working in your life, you should actively look for ways to change. However, you don't want this self-assessment to turn into self-recrimination. You don't want to lower your self-esteem. A good self-assessment means coaching yourself in positive ways to find answers that are really going to assist you on life's journey. Become solution oriented every step of the way.

Let's take a look at three trouble spots that many of us experience. Let's say that you are in the habit of telling yourself:

- **"I would do a lot of things if only I had the time."** All of us would like to have more time in our schedules. But spare hours are relatively hard to find. If you wait for large chunks of time, *you will fall further behind* in your efforts each week.

  Instead, learn to use small bits of time. As we have mentioned in previous chapters, a few minutes used to make an important phone call or to find out a piece of information adds up.

  Here's a new habit to try: Do one small thing each day *that will make a difference a year from now.* For example, make a phone call to schedule yourself for a computer spreadsheets class. If you attend, you probably will reap rewards one year from now—and beyond.

Or, take five minutes to learn something important from your supervisor. If the information is truly enlightening, it will help you one year from now. It may even help you ten years from now.

- **"Other people are always pulling me off course—messing up my goals."** This is an easy trap to fall into. Other people probably *do* need attention from you constantly. But learn to govern and protect your personal time.

  There will always be someone who knowingly or inadvertently steals time from your agenda. This person may deliberately tie up your valuable time for his or her own selfish needs or may simply need your assistance too much. Be vigilant that you guard against those who interfere with your goals.

  Here's a new habit to try: Practice carving out time in which you can work or play without being disturbed. Start with small amounts of time, even 10 or 15 minutes. Then gradually work up to an hour or two. Practice setting the boundary verbally with others that you are not to be interrupted.

  As you teach others about your need for personal time, they will come to accept it more fully. They will believe you're serious about your boundary *when you become serious about it.*

  Try this additional self-help measure: Refrain from announcing your goals to those who would sabotage your plans. For example, if you want to spend an afternoon alone walking through downtown shops, don't inform your friends—who may instantly volunteer to come along with several children in tow. Sometimes the best boundary is to just keep quiet.

  If others constantly throw you off course, ask yourself, "Do I set myself up for failure?" Maybe you're too flexible, too open about sharing information, or too accommodating for your own good.

- **"I have too many things in my life that are draining me. I can't make any progress."** Any individual could find a hundred negative things to ponder. If you dwell on problems, without a direct plan of action, *you will begin to drain your own energies.* You must change some personal habits in order to stop giving away your personal power.

  Here's a new habit to try: Put a time limit on your worries. For example, if you spend a lot of time reflecting on the shortcomings of others, allow yourself 10 minutes per day for that piece of business. Then *force yourself* to focus on something else.

  Do you spend a lot of time worrying over station politics or stressful scenes which have upset you? Carve out a certain period of time each day to mull these things over. Then either make a plan for handling the situation, or force yourself to focus on something else.

Changing habits involves a huge amount of willpower. Clever tricks and self-help plans can never take the place of good old-fashioned willpower. Exercising willpower is all part of the package of becoming your best self. The payoffs are many, however.

For instance, when you faithfully work on self-improvement, a negative past cannot *control you* anymore. It may still *bother you* in certain ways, but it cannot control you anymore. When you focus strongly on achievement and reaching goals, you'll be moving yourself forward into a better future where negative experiences will lose their hold on you.

Coming to terms with an extremely stressful past—a bad childhood or an ugly divorce—is *never easy.* It involves some of the most challenging work known to humankind. But no matter what has happened to you, you can rise above it. You cannot change what has happened, of course. Even through your best efforts, you may never feel terrific about your past. But you can learn to leave it alone *by moving past it.* You do this when you actively work to *move into a more productive future.*

It is never wise to say, "I'll just forget the past." If there are problem areas in your past, you need to thoroughly assess what has transpired. In fact, you may need assistance from friends or a counselor in dealing with certain issues. But while you're working through the stress—or even intense pain—*always hold yourself accountable for self-improvement.* If you have been hurt by the past, you owe it to yourself to create a better future.

> *"Last summer, I ran into an old high school chum," says Lydia, a paramedic from the West. "She'd been dumped by her husband seven years earlier. When I asked her if she'd remarried, she looked at me kind of sheepishly.*
>
> *"My friend said, 'No, I'm not remarried. We're still working out the details of the divorce. It's supposed to come up in court next month.'*
>
> *"Now, I may not be the most ambitious person on earth," says Lydia, "but if my husband had dumped me seven years ago, I'd be well into a new life by now. I might not be remarried, but I'd have that chapter closed."*

In assessing your personal approach to problems, make sure that you are not getting stuck in neutral. You need to stay in touch with all of those things that keep you from succeeding. *Continually coach yourself* toward getting around those roadblocks.

As you practice self-empowerment, remember to treat yourself with kindness. Decide to be your own best friend. How you communicate with yourself is instrumental in relieving stress as you go along in life. Those messages you give yourself can make the difference between making progress and sinking into a depression.

For instance, do you refrain from berating yourself when things aren't going well? Do you patiently steer yourself toward goals? Are you good at assessing your options calmly?

If you're not happy with a certain situation, you can improve it without beating yourself up or judging yourself too harshly. By exercising small measures of control, you will learn to build self-confidence. You will learn what you can and cannot do. None of us can do everything. We don't have that kind of power. But we can do *what's important.* We can choose enough options to bring harmony to our lives.

In order to create more harmony in your life, you need to trust your "inner voice." When your stress levels are high, review your choices and then *look inward for the answers you need.* You are the best expert on yourself. Ultimately, you know what will work for you in a personal situation.

These suggestions can help you propel yourself in the direction you want to go:

- **Take time to define what a balanced life means.** Have you taken the time to get in touch with what daily agenda or lifestyle would feel harmonious to you?

    You may be struggling to define what it is because you're trying to copy someone else's goals or lifestyle. If you crave a simple lifestyle in a cottage by the lake, don't vary from this basic concept. Stick to your own definition of success.

- **Believe you can do anything that you really want to do.** Why? Because you will start to *focus your power.* You won't feel as confused. You won't be torn between various choices.

    Also, having faith that you can accomplish your heart's desire gives you a sense of certainty. *This confidence will attract what you need.* Notice how other people will start helping you *when they're convinced you're serious* about achieving a goal.

    There is nothing so attractive as a confident person who knows exactly what he or she wants. People enjoy contributing to a confident person's plan because they feel their contributions or suggestions have an excellent chance of being utilized.

    All of us enjoy having strong, confident friends who know how to reach goals. When we assist them, *we are part of them,* and they become part of us. That's how each of us builds a support system.

- **Do you motivate yourself in the right ways?** For instance, do you remind yourself of *why* you are pushing toward certain goals? What are you after?

    Tell yourself why you're taking a class or running at 6:30 A.M. when some people are still in bed. Motivation must be fed into your psyche on a continual basis. Don't give yourself a pep talk once a week. Do it every day.

Assess yourself as a whole person

When you become the captain of your ship, and take responsibility for every single area of your life, you will feel more congruency in your life. You will feel more complete and less fragmented.

"You cannot separate the different areas of your life," says Chuck Burkell, program chair of the executive development curriculum at the National Fire Academy in Emmitsburg, Maryland.

Burkell, who has assisted many men and women on the EMS–fire career ladder, believes emergency responders should actively seek feedback from their peers in making a career plan or a life plan. "What helps is to find coworkers who'll help you assess your strengths and weaknesses," he emphasizes.

Although you want to solicit help from *supportive* coworkers, it can still be scary to assess yourself. It also can be very unsettling to look one of your friends in the eye and say, "Help me figure out what I'm doing wrong." But if you feel stuck, you're only going to get unstuck if you face the truth.

For example, could your attitude be better? Do you put yourself down? Do you act unsure in certain situations where a more confident attitude would be beneficial? Are you associating with people who are dragging you down? Do you try to pursue too many goals at once—only to end up dropping your efforts totally?

A supportive friend can hold a mirror up to you. In this mirror, you will see mistakes. But don't identify with these mistakes in an overly personal way. You can

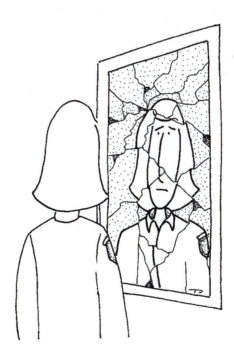

change most of them. These mistakes do not have to be part of your permanent persona—unless you fail to correct them. They are only small rocks in your path.

Removing them can be an enjoyable experience. Every time you remove a small obstacle, attain a new habit, or correct some unfortunate situation in your life, you are empowering yourself to do better, feel better, and even look more attractive.

> *"A friend can be objective in helping you reduce stress," says Trish, a vice captain at an urban fire–EMS station. "When you've lived under a tremendous amount of stress for a long time, you can lose touch with a large part of yourself. I looked in the mirror one morning, and I didn't recognize myself. I looked kind of numb and expressionless. I have to say, I didn't look attractive at all.*
>
> *"I'd been living under so much stress for two or three years, that something in me was dead. I needed to be revived. My job is hectic, and so is my personal life. I felt frozen in one spot like a robot required to perform one task over and over."*
>
> *She continues, "You get to the point in life where you'd like something great to happen. You'd like to look better and feel better—feel good, feel alive. But you just sit around waiting—and it never comes."*

Trish's best friend helped her assess three areas of her life. She told Trish, "You need to give yourself a break." With the best of intentions, Trish was throwing her life out of balance by expecting too much of herself. She did curtail a lot of her self-defeat by making these changes:

- She stopped robbing herself of sleep.

  > *"I had this bad habit of seeing how much I could do in a given day," says Trish. I'd jump around answering the phone while I cooked dinner. I'd write notes and try to e-mail simultaneously. I stuck notes all over my car. When bedtime came, I'd be reading two magazines and flossing my teeth.*
  >
  > *"I finally decided that my batteries were so low that nothing was going to change until I found a few extra hours of sleep each week. So now, I don't care if the dishes are piled high in the sink. As long as the kids are okay, I fall into bed and give myself permission to sleep."*

- She solicited support in caring for her aging parents.

  > *"I found a social worker who calls to check in with my parents on a daily basis," says Trish. "They live in another city. Having this social worker involved gives me a little added support. My parents feel good about it, too.*
  >
  > *"There is nothing like the pressure of thinking your parents are sick or in trouble—and you're living in another city," she emphasizes.*

- She made two changes in her routine.

"First, I started jogging 45 minutes three times a week. I used to do aerobics, but I needed a different kind of workout. I like moving through the streets with all of that freedom. I use the running time to think and plan.

"Second, I've hired my teenage daughter to shop for groceries every other weekend. The driving to and from the store, shopping, and then putting the groceries away kills my entire morning. I pay my daughter fifteen dollars each time," says Trish. "She speeds through the store in half the time it would take me. She's learning good life skills and seems happy with the job. I can't afford to pay her every week, but two weekends per month works fine."

In creating harmony in your life, it helps to utilize the resources you have—however small they may seem. For instance, could you ask a neighbor to help move three boxes of junk out of your basement? Would taking healthy foods to work help you feel better and have more energy?

Some people, however, seem to thrive on chaos instead of productive self-help. Focusing on chaos instead of productivity is not only counterproductive, it can be *addictive*. Thinking about chaos can give you an adrenaline rush.

Reminder

If you are a codependent personality type, you can become *addicted to focusing on chaos* in order to feel emotionally charged. But this habit can waste precious hours of your life. You have only a finite amount of mental and emotional energy in a single day. When that's gone, you've spent the fuel you needed to improve your life.

"I used to sit around the station listening to negative conversations," says Pam, a first responder. "I thrived on these pity parties. Hearing other people's relationship problems or financial troubles made mine not seem so bad.

"But I finally woke up," she asserts. "I knew I needed to cut these conversations short. I started working out in the station workout room. I started studying more, figuring out a few goals, and trying to turn my life around. I'm now twenty pounds lighter. I'm getting more organized. And I'm slowly, but surely completing the coursework to become a paramedic."

Whenever you feel frustrated, it helps to do a self-assessment of how you're spending your time. Work to uncover any counterproductive routines. Figure out what's stealing your energy, your attention, and ultimately, your future. Take a careful look at how you manage your responsibilities.

Reflect on questions such as these:

- Is there a situation in your life that you're not dealing with constructively? Maybe you keep pushing it out of your mind.

- Do you need to reach out for some kind of help, but you are letting pride stop you?

- Do you spend too much time on the telephone?

- Are you languishing in conversations that are counterproductive?

- Do you have certain fears—even phobias—that are hindering your career or personal success?

As you look at how you're handling your life, keep in mind that fear is a major area to address. Fear is sometimes the stumbling block for finding relief for your stress.

For example, Hayden, a young paramedic, did not feel comfortable in social situations. He just couldn't keep a conversation rolling like some people could. This affected his dating. "And ultimately," says Hayden, "it was affecting my mating. I couldn't find the right girl if I couldn't bring myself to socialize.

"I really was phobic about social settings," he continues. "But finally I made a plan for self-help. I cured myself of my social anxieties. By the way, I do have a significant other, and we're getting closer to becoming engaged."

Hayden did the following to overcome his social shyness:

- He forced himself to speak to two strangers every day.

  "The checkout girl at the corner convenience store was my starting point," he says.

- He took an interest in all of his neighbors.

  "I live in a safe apartment building, so I made myself strike up conversations with others," he stresses. "I offered help in carrying groceries or in any way I could."

- He joined a church group where he would have to interact.

  "We meet for dinner once a week. It became easy to chat with these people because they took such a personal interest in me," he explains.

Conquering a fear can be scary. Trying to end the fear—or at least tame it down somewhat—means you're going to have to take some type of risk. But if risks are well-planned and carefully calculated, they can yield good payoffs. Taking risks can improve the quality of your life.

Taking a risk in a personal situation

"I'm a divorced father," says Zak, who works for an emergency training center. "My ex-wife was always giving me a hard time about our child. This woman's mission in life was to make me pay—financially and emotionally. I dreaded answering the phone. I approached her father, my ex-father-in-law, to ask him if he'd act as mediator for relaying our conversations. I knew he was a fair guy whom I could trust.

"I was taking a risk in asking him to help. He could have said no. He could have perceived me as weak. But all I can say is, the risk worked. I don't deal directly with my ex-wife anymore. She knows she has to communicate with me through her father. This might not work for anyone else, but it turned out to be all that saved my sanity."

AN ATTITUDE ADJUSTMENT

Although you don't want to control others in a negative way—or become obsessive about getting your own way all of the time—you do want to find control that puts you in the driver's seat of your destiny. Sometimes, a control button is something as simple as developing a better attitude.

"I used to feel sorry for myself a lot when I was in the military," says Jason, a paramedic who began his career as a Navy medic. "I found fault with the world and everybody in it. At 28, I thought life was passing me by. I needed a real attitude adjustment. One spring day, I found a great teacher."

He continues, "I had been dispatched to a nursing home on a Veterans Affairs Campus to pick up medical records. One of the male nurses asked me, 'Would you like to meet the oldest veteran in the state?'

"The nurse led me into a room where this 103-year-old man greeted me with open arms. He was a good looking man—nice hair, smooth skin, and well-groomed. Didn't look past his late seventies. He told me he was grateful for the care he was receiving. He was glad to be alive. Said he couldn't wait for the dogwood trees outside to bloom.

"I sat down on the edge of the bed. I started asking him everything—whom he'd married, where he worked, what branch of the service he'd been in. After about 10 minutes into the conversation, he said, 'My two nephews are coming later to play cards with me.'

"Do you have any children?" I inquired. 'No, I don't. But that could happen,' he said. Then he tapped me playfully and added, 'My life's not over yet.' "

A good attitude is the oil of life. It will reduce friction as you manage stressful situations. A good attitude will affect the quality of your work, the quality of your relationships, and ultimately your own mental and physical well-being. It will give you a vibrancy that enhances your attractiveness to others. It will give you a social and professional edge that nothing else can.

You will feel more balance in life when you operate from a position of personal strength. You also will feel stronger when you're striving to reach your full potential. It is easier to make stress work *for you* when you take this approach. Why? When you focus on the payoffs, you'll perceive the pressures as all part of the game.

Also, you're going to feel more personally grounded when you take pride in your daily activities. This pride activates the mental fuel you need to feed your ego. Think of your ego as your *spirit*. Never become egotistical, but do everything you can to feel good about yourself. You want to do impressive work, and you want to help others do the same.

Also, in order to empower yourself, you must clue in on what is going on around you. It can be very self-defeating if you fail to read other people accurately. For example, learn others' weaknesses so you won't get caught up in those weaknesses. If you are associating with people who aren't going to be supportive of you, you need to know that early on.

Being your best self will require that you handle a lot of stress issues *before* they arise. For example, quickly finding clues about the shortcomings of others will serve as a form of personal protection for you. Although you never want to use other people's weaknesses against them, you must become wise to the personal habits of those around you. Their foibles and follies can easily hurt your success. Your goal is to hurt no one. But you must learn to protect your own interests in every possible way.

"I could have been promoted three years ago, but I thought it would upset my friends," says Milton, a newly appointed lieutenant at a fire station. "I finally took the promotion, and it did upset them. They acted differently toward me, and their jealousies took the form of all kinds of snide remarks. One of my so-called friends finally quit his job. He was in the wrong field. And the other man got fired for coming in late so often.

"I'll never ask other people's permission to excel again," he laughs. "That was some kind of weird weakness in me. I'm now comfortable with the fact that every choice I make might displease someone."

Needing the approval of others too much will throw your life off balance. It certainly can stifle your career advancement. You should learn to validate your own decisions and know if they are good ones. Constantly coach yourself to believe that you can trust yourself in difficult situations. *Never* doubt your own instincts. Sometimes it isn't wise to act on instinct alone, but pay attention to your deepest feelings when you have nothing else to rely on.

By coaching yourself to do well under pressure, you can feel less stress in a critical triage situation or in a major disaster. When you talk to yourself in supportive ways, you will waste less energy on worry and nonsense. You will learn to go into the heat of battle—managing a multistory fire or striving to locate a child lost in the woods—with true focus. By focusing well on each moment of your life, you don't have to spend too much time doubting yourself or second-guessing your abilities.

BECOME GOAL ORIENTED

When you work toward a better career or a better personal life, you'll need to set definitive goals. Goals give our lives purpose and direction. They shape and define our lives. But goals can *increase* your stress levels if you have either too few or too many of them. Either extreme will make you feel out of control. Practice setting the right amount of goals for yourself. Always err on the side of setting too few goals, until you become adept at structuring and reaching goals.

Write down each goal. Visualize that goal by really seeing it as part of your reality. See yourself in the picture, happy that you have arrived at your destination. What does it look like? What does it feel like? How much happiness does it bring you? What are the benefits? The risks? Are you willing to fight for it?

When you become emotionally involved with a goal, it becomes a part of you. It seems more real. It demands attention. Keep in mind the following points for reaching goals. Ask yourself:

- **Am I an expert at setting small goals?** When you feel confident that you can reach lots of small goals, it is just a matter of time before you can take bigger steps. In order to improve the quality of your life, there will be times when you must make larger leaps to get what you want. By tackling lots of small goals and watching them come to fruition, you will be in a better position to know if you can make larger plans materialize.

- **Am I connected to my support?** It is much easier to work toward goals if you have people in your life who are encouraging you. Without encouragement, it's very difficult to keep going when the pressure is on. Sometimes it helps tremendously to call a friend for five minutes to get a daily pep talk. If you're trying to finish a course or land a new job, the effort can seem lonely without knowing that at least one person is cheering for you to succeed. Having supportive people also provides, in a positive way, individuals to hold you accountable *if you fail to arrive* at your desired goals.

- **Do I allow myself to run out of options?** Always keep in mind that every task has more than one solution or method for completion, excepting precise medical skills for helping a patient. Naturally, you can't change predetermined protocols on the job. But do figure at least two or three ways to accomplish a task for coordinating others or taking better care of your family. Never get in the habit of believing there's only one way to make something happen. This can make you feel very victimized when things don't run smoothly.

- **Do I take into account the feelings of those close to me?** For example, if you want to move to Milwaukee but your spouse prefers a warm climate year-round, you might need to reconsider your options. Your job and your personal life must work as a whole. It will be hard for those in your support system to back your plans if you don't fully consider their feelings.

In order to ensure that a goal will materialize, it helps to ask yourself a few questions such as:

- What price will I pay personally or professionally *if I fail to take control?*
- How can I make a plan to implement change?
- What are the obstacles standing in my way?
- How can I remove those obstacles?

As you work toward your goals, you must learn to manage yourself in ways that conserve your energy. Be a stickler for spending your mental and physical energies wisely. Use these strategies for taking good care of yourself:

- **Give enough to others to feel good about yourself.** *Then stop.* If you don't have healthy boundaries that separate you from other people, you will begin to resent those people. Anyone in a helping profession—including emergency responders, doctors, nurses, or psychologists—must learn to maintain a cutoff point in worrying about, giving to, grieving for, or rescuing others.

- **Put responsibility back onto the plates of others.** Balance comes from doing your share in all things—and doing these things willingly and gracefully—but do not falsely accept responsibility that belongs to others.

- **Don't forget that knowledge is power.** It will take much longer to reach any goal if you lack information about the steps for making it happen. Education, both formal and informal, is instrumental in bringing balance to your life. If you feel out of control in making some of your

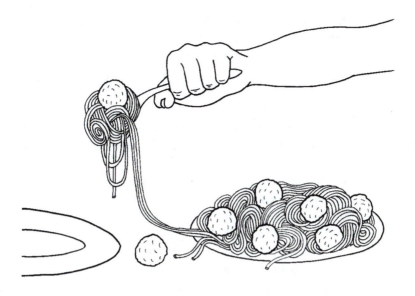

most important goals materialize, you probably need more education in certain areas.

SELF-ASSESSMENT IN THE WORK ARENA

If you want to feel more balance at work, take a look at how your being passive can hurt you. What are you doing, if anything, to trip yourself up? Are you wasting time trying to get promoted where the opportunities are limited? Are you blaming yourself unfairly when you need to educate yourself about the *total picture* of your workplace setting?

Reducing your stress becomes easier when you comprehend the true picture. You won't be wasting time trying to open doors that won't open. You can make alternative plans.

If you fully understand the total picture around you, you will know which goals are worth pursuing in your work arena. You can assess how to become your personal best in your present situation without striving to change the impossible.

Assessing yourself properly can help you work smarter. You can quickly reverse self-defeating patterns in the workplace when you understand the way around certain roadblocks. In order to empower yourself in your career, consider these questions:

- **Have you learned part of the job above you?** This must be done covertly, of course. Be discreet about understanding certain tasks your supervisor must perform. After all, you don't want to be perceived as competition for your boss. But by knowing your supervisor's problems, you will know how to be a better worker. You will know how to enhance your role in *appropriate* ways.

- **Have you created a niche for yourself?** Figure out the stress factors of your supervisors and try to help them fix their problems. By offering to relieve stress for others, you will be acquiring the best job insurance you'll ever have. Even if your company has layoffs or folds completely, you'll have supervisors who will recommend you to other employers.

- **Could you learn your job more thoroughly by teaching skills to others?** By showing others how to excel, you will excel. If you want to supervise others or teach one day, you need to start practicing now. No one attains great teaching skills overnight. It takes years of practice. By sharing your knowledge, you will learn the best ways to convey information. By stimulating the minds of those around you, you are adding information to your own educational bank.

- **Do you have a clue about the true problems of management?** If not, do your homework. By knowing the inside scoop of what's going on, you can decide *how much of your career* you are willing to devote to your department. Whether you stay or leave, you want to make either decision based on sound knowledge. When you actively pay attention to the problems of those supervising you, your own role in the department should become clearer.

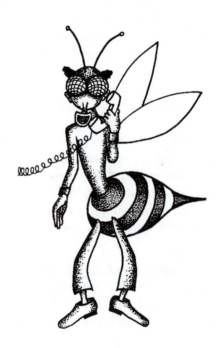

"I used to work for a small private EMS company where the budget was very in-adequate," says Scott, a firefighter–paramedic who has assisted architects in de-signing new fire stations.

"At this station, the employees were always after the boss for a raise. I've always been a realist, so I knew there wasn't going to be a raise. I knew I'd have to get hired at a county EMS service to get more benefits and more pay."

He continues, *"When I finally landed a job with the county service, there were men and women I'd worked with at the private service who acted shocked that I'd landed my new job. They asked me what kind of political strings I'd pulled. They just knew I'd done something dishonest to sneak myself up the ladder one little notch.*

"I hadn't pulled any strings," Scott insists. *"I just had a résumé on file with the county which I'd crafted with precision. I called back every week to make a pest of myself,"* he laughs. *"I let the county administrators know I meant business about getting hired. You don't have to plan a lot of moves to get anywhere. You just have to carefully plan your* next *move."*

NAVIGATIONAL TOOLS

People who have ever attained success have been confused at some point. They had to figure out how to get through the woods. Those who succeed in life must blaze a trail. This can be fearful. Pushing ahead without a map is difficult. Anyone who leaves a comfortable, known environment to push ahead to unknown territory is go-ing to take some scrapes and bruises. It takes discipline to keep going.

If you believe that it's hard to discipline yourself to accomplish what you want to do, just try coping with the stress of *not taking control.* For one thing, you will be at the mercy of other people's decisions a good deal of the time.

Even if you are 45 or 50, you should always pay close attention to your career needs and personal needs. You can forget that younger, talented people are always pushing for your job. You can forget to nurture your personal relationships. One day, if you don't pay attention, you may wake up to find your relationships or your career in a crisis situation.

"I went through a painful divorce at 50," says Johnny, a retired fire chief. *"Di-vorce is a real shock to a 50-year-old's system. I had to get a plan going, and cre-ating a plan for your life at this age is challenging. It's not like making a plan to finish a basic ACLS course. A plan for your life has no syllabus. You have to write that plan yourself. But if you fail to write it, someone else or something else will write it for you."*

Johnny has since remarried and he's on good terms with his ex-wife. *"I won't say that getting to the point I'm at now was easy,"* he explains. *"It wasn't. Starting over feels terrible in a lot of ways. You feel that a lot of your life was wasted. But when you make up your mind to improve yourself and become better, instead of bitter, you'll make it. Life offers a lot of good things every day. You just have to tell yourself that you'll reach out for more. That's how you turn a crisis around."*

Successful, happy individuals have certain traits in common. They strive to be upbeat and work hard to attain the goals that are important to them. In addition, they learn to program themselves to expect good things from life. If you want to be a happier person, try these techniques for managing your life:

- **Live only 24 hours at a time.** Try to avoid worrying about yesterday's problems or tomorrow's problems. Just focus on doing well today.

- **Be grateful for what you have.** Happy individuals constantly reflect on all of the things they have to be thankful for. In fact, without this attitude, it's practically impossible to be happy. A feeling of gratitude is always the basis for wanting to do more. Keep reminding yourself of what you have achieved and how far you have come.

- **Study other productive people but never envy them.** Learning all you can about how others manage their time or their lives is productive. But comparing yourself to others isn't. Much unhappiness can result from comparing yourself unfavorably to other people. Each of us must walk an individual path, so don't waste time wishing you were in someone else's shoes.

  "I used to envy my brother-in-law a lot," says Denver, an ex-Marine who is now in paramedic school. "He had a sailboat. He took trips to Alaska. But when I started being more grateful for my own life, I felt more at peace. I started reflecting on how lucky I am to have a strong body. I count my blessings that I can get out and bike or run. I have two beautiful children.

  "We all have more assets than we think we do. We just forget to notice them when we're caught up in being busy. The perfect way to double all of your assets is to be twice as thankful for what you already have."

REVIEW ACTIVITIES

1. List three goals you'd like to attain in the next six months. Break them down into steps to figure out how you can achieve them.

2. Why is it important to believe you can do anything you really want to do?

3. Name two areas of your life that are causing you stress. How could you possibly relieve the stress in these areas by changing something within yourself?

4. Name two habits you'd like to change in the near future. What type of plan would you need for acquiring new habits to replace the old?

5. Describe a situation where you increased your stress levels by getting caught up in the negative conversations of other people. How would you handle that same situation now?

6. Why is it unproductive to do the absolute minimum to get by? What do you think would happen if you applied this approach to many of your tasks?

7. Name three ways that having a good attitude can improve one's life.

8. List two people whose work habits are impressive. What could you learn by studying the methods of these people?

FOR SUPERVISORS

1. You are concerned that someone you supervise has a self-discipline problem. How could you help this person work toward self-control? For example, can you think of small steps this individual could take to improve his or her self-discipline? Name five reasons why self-discipline actually makes anyone's work easier in the long run.

2. Let's say that your future goal is to become an EMS state administrator. Name one personal weakness that could interfere with your reaching this goal. Name three personal strengths you now possess that could definitely help you reach this goal.

CLASS PROJECT

1. Appoint three groups of people with four individuals to a group. Name one person in each group to create his or her career plan. Have the others in the group guide the selected individual. Have the ones doing the mentoring write good self-assessment questions for the individual making the plan. Have the class vote on the best career plan of the three groups.

CHAPTER TEN

WRITING A CAREER PLAN–LIFE PLAN

Do you dream of owning your own ambulance service someday? Or would you enjoy teaching EMS? Maybe you'd like to write textbooks, reference books, or training materials for EMTs and paramedics. You can accomplish most of your dreams if you take the right steps. How successful you become, whether in terms of a paycheck or personal happiness, will depend largely on how well you plan.

Your planning does not need to be a lengthy undertaking. You can write notes, lists, and goals in any fashion that makes sense to you. But it does help to get your plan on paper. Having information in writing will help you to track your progress. You can hold yourself accountable for following through on changes you need to implement.

It is helpful to create both a career plan and a plan for your *personal life*. A good plan is like having a road map for guiding your journey. A good map makes any trip less stressful. The more specific you make your plan, the more likely your chances of hitting your desired "targets" or goals.

Have you ever bought items to decorate your home without working from a plan? Perhaps you purchased lamps or rugs on sale—only to discover that your purchases didn't really fit your décor. They clashed with your color scheme. You lost time by having to exchange those items. Or, you ended up losing money by failing to return them. Your lamps and rugs wound up in a yard sale. Or, you actually used your new items—only to feel dissatisfied every time you looked at them. Had you started with a plan, your efforts would have been more productive.

Proper planning for your personal or professional life will guarantee that more of your efforts will fit into a grand scheme. For example, every self-improvement class you take or every skill you acquire can harmonize with your larger ambitions. Having the right people in your planning process can help, too. Always record phone numbers, addresses, and e-mail addresses quickly in your notebook. Tiny bits of paper and business cards can get lost. You never know when someone you meet today can help you tomorrow. But people can't help you unless you keep track of who they are and where to locate them.

"I used to feel like I was trapped in the spin cycle of a washing machine," says Derrick, a 39-year-old paramedic. "I was so busy working two EMS jobs that I couldn't plan anything. I was too exhausted to think about making any changes in my life or in my career.

"My boss was intrigued about a career planning seminar that was coming to our city. He asked me to go with him. I think it cost $125. I didn't want to tell him I couldn't really afford to spend money like this. So I scrounged up the money and went. I sat through this seminar, just seeing the lightbulbs come on. I saw that I had choices.

"I was exhausted working two intense jobs, because I had not taken control of my choices. I started laying groundwork for the job I have now. I work with an air ambulance service. I'm not exhausted. I'm having the time of my life, and I make enough money to live well. Planning is all that got me here."

Here are some areas to think about in writing a career plan or a life plan:

- What are your long-term goals?
- What are your short-term goals?
- What obstacles or "roadblocks" are preventing you from reaching those goals?

"My long-term goal is to own an EMS-related products supply business one day," says Kerry, a firefighter–paramedic. "I think about this all the time. I love EMS, and I enjoy the business world, so this career goal would be the perfect blend. My main obstacle to reaching this goal is that I need investment capital. So I started networking with members of investment clubs in my community and two invest-ment bankers.

"Some of my friends have said, 'Kerry, you'll never be able to compete with the com-panies that are already out there. You're dreaming.' Well, somebody has to dream. My part in this is to develop the skills I need. I'm keeping a file on supplies needed for our local EMS stations which I could buy from a large wholesaler. I'm asking a lot of questions and talking with people who have started their own businesses. If I concentrate on what service I want to deliver, I'll locate the start-up money."

Believing that you can achieve something is the starting point, of course. If you act confident about achieving your goal, speak confidently to others who might help you, and research information as if you plan to succeed, you will get the wheels turning.

How Do You Start?

Your written career plan can be as simple as keeping two or three pages of notes. Or, it can be a very detailed, even lengthy, undertaking. Although you don't need to overburden yourself by including too much, the more detailed you can make your plan, the better.

Writing your own program for career advancement—whether you use a composition notebook or computer software—means devising a goal-oriented plan. By breaking the goals down into categories, you will be able to keep track of your progress. This plan should have categories for every area you want to improve or change.

Your major goals should include all of the steps needed to "conquer" them. Every small step you outline should support your larger plans. Every large goal should excite you. It is much easier to climb a ladder, rung by rung, if you're eager to reach the top. Because enthusiasm is a key ingredient for reaching any goal, it will probably be more productive to make loftier goals rather than average ones. There's something about an average goal that doesn't demand too much attention. An average goal can sit on a mental shelf and collect dust.

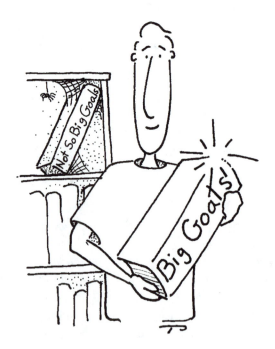

By feeling truly excited about your goals, you will be willing to sacrifice more time and energy to ensure their completion. You'll be willing to stay focused, do the small steps of your plan, and get to work *sooner,* rather than later.

Having a plan for your life and your career will demand that you do enough research to stay abreast of the job market. By researching choices, you'll figure out that there is always more than one direction to go. Writing a plan, complete with many options for employment, can help to stabilize your career through company buyouts and career shakeups. When you run out of ideas, you will soon discover, through planning, that there's always one more good idea you hadn't previously considered.

> *"I've changed employers three times in my 25-year career," says Cal, an EMT from rural Iowa. "On job losses, I received little notice I was going to be unemployed. While I've never been out of work for long, I've had to think up clever strategies to find a new job.*
>
> *"If you love EMS as much as I do, you'll plot and scheme to stay in this line of work," he laughs. "When I lost my last job, I called all of the people in my professional network. No one knew of a job. So I began to call people outside of my network.*
>
> *"I remembered a CPR class I'd taught for a railroad office in a nearby town. I had the main boss's private number and pager number in my personal planner. I dialed him up to see if he might know of a job. I introduced myself and said, 'Do you remember me, by any chance?'*
>
> *"He said, 'Yes, I do. The class you taught saved my baby grandson's life. My wife and I were babysitting and he stopped breathing. I had to do CPR on him, and I did it exactly the way you explained for infants. I blew gently, like blowing out a candle.'*
>
> *"I then blustered out something about needing to find a job. Then I started to hang up. But the man said, 'Hold on. There's a rescue squad right across from our yard office. I'll call them to see if they need anyone.' Well, they did and I was hired within three weeks. To top things off, I've been paid to teach dozens of CPR classes for railroad employees.*
>
> *"I don't mean to imply that you should capitalize on people you've helped, but you do need to think of everyone to call when you have a real need. I hate to think what might have happened if I'd lost that railroad administrator's number. One contact can open many doors."*

As you work on your long-term career plan or your next job move, be inventive. Consider all possible trails to blaze—even if some of the alternatives don't comply with your immediate desires. By finding more alternatives, you can create the work style and lifestyle that harmonize with your needs, your talents, and your personal preferences.

For example, you might want to work as an EMT while supplementing your income with a craft or trade. Or, you might want to become a police officer cross-trained in EMS who teaches safety courses at local businesses for a fee. As an EMS firefighter, you might decide that owning a small family business with your spouse fits into your plans. That way, you and your spouse will have a common interest.

Consider these strategies for evaluating more alternatives:

- **Think in terms of being an entrepreneur.** Rest assured that you have more marketable skills than you'd first think. It is crucial to sell those skills in the right way. Ponder many ways to market yourself. For example, Taylor, a paramedic who also works part time in an ER felt he could earn extra cash by conducting a public speaking seminar at a local hospital.

  He had been in a speech club since his freshman year in high school. His oral presentation skills were excellent. He had learned through networking that lots of hospital staff, including several doctors, needed coaching in how to give oral presentations.

  "I make $200 an hour teaching five one-hour classes per month," he says. "Some of my students do not have a clue about organizing a speech. They are brilliant professionally, but they need help on altering their voice tones throughout a speech, gesturing correctly, and polishing their overall platform skills.

  "What's gratifying is that one surgeon asked me to coach him, video his talks, and help him prepare for speaking at a conference. I worked with him for four months to help him polish his presentation. When he spoke at his conference, he was so proud of himself, he called me from the opposite coast to say 'Thank you.' "

- **Keep your priorities straight.** Pursue what you value most in life. The only reason people do not reach their goals is that they allow themselves to become sidetracked. There will *always* be something pulling you away from your goals. But persevere to stay on course.

The more precisely you plan, the more chances you'll have to work in harmony with what's important to you. Money is always part of the picture, but it should not be the whole picture. Some of your goals should have nothing to do with financial gain. A good plan will give you the incentive to try more things that truly interest you.

- **Daydreaming is extremely important.** It helps mentally to create situations you want to materialize. You can certainly create a fuzzy career picture—and a lifestyle to match. But who wants that? Use your imagination to put in all of the glorious details.

    Let's say that your dream is to work in management for an EMS county division in Texas. Texas is your native state, but you've been working in Pennsylvania for five years. Your desire is to return to the South. In your spare time, you'd like to raise horses and paint landscapes. If you make your goals that precise, your subconscious mind will start helping you. You'll start to notice job ads, people, and opportunities connected with Texas.

Visualizing where you want to be three years from now, or fifteen years from now, should always include an abundance of details about the work environment you'd enjoy, the kinds of people you would like to meet, the type of home life you want, and the kind of daily routine that would feel best to you.

Why will visualizing help? Because it's hard to believe you can reach any goal if you can't see yourself physically connected to it. It will seem too foreign—like it could happen to someone else, but not to you. Visualizing helps you have the faith to keep going when your dream is threatened by setbacks, a personal illness, or financial problems. Few people have reached major goals without detours. But seeing yourself arriving at your desired destination is important for *keeping the faith* that you'll get there.

> "Some of my friends have laughed at me," says Jane, an EMT. "I've quit EMS three times in the last five years. But I've always returned! I love being an EMT, but I've had upheavals in my personal life. I've also been affected by a major family illness.
>
> "My career planning has been nonexistent. I've not been very good at picturing what I want and that's probably why I'm off track. But I want to take control of that. There comes a point in your life when you get so frustrated. It's draining to be lost on a career track—even if it's unavoidable. I want to get on the straight and narrow. My dream would be to work in EMS management. My goal this year is to take one office management class. It doesn't sound like much, but I have to start somewhere."

Getting down to business

In order to begin your career plan–life plan, write down at least three long-term goals and three short-term goals you want to reach. Make sure that your short-term goals support your long-term ones. When you write goals down, you can come back to fine-tune them later.

For example, you could begin like this:

My long-term goals are:

1. To become a paramedic instructor
2. To serve on a state EMS advisory committee
3. To build a house for my family

Your short-term goals might include offering to teach two classes per month for local training sessions to support your number-one goal. Another short-term goal might be to ask your supervisor how an individual might earn the privilege to sit on an advisory committee. For example, should you write a letter to someone? Should you attend an open meeting of that committee?

On your goal to build a house, one short-term goal might be to meet with two individuals who could quote a price for a complete home package. Another goal might be to check out prices on lots in a new subdivision that appeals to you. Yet another might be to meet with one or two mortgage lenders to discuss interest rates and other information.

Keep in mind that with any type of planning it will be your *skills* that push your goals forward. *Skills really are your leverage in making things happen.* In order to become a paramedic instructor, for instance, you can't just have medical skills and teaching skills. You must have the skills to sell yourself in a job interview. You also need skills for negotiating a salary, skills for planning your teaching syllabus, and skills for upgrading your teaching abilities on a regular basis.

Skills always give you confidence, too. Confidence can be the very foundation of winning the prize you want. Remember that you need just as many skills in your personal life as you do in your professional life. Research, education, networking, and planning are skills that will benefit your family. For example, Ellen, a 28-year-old newly married EMT, attained home ownership by skillfully researching her options and then acting with confidence.

"My husband and I wanted to buy a new house," says Ellen. "We couldn't afford a dream house but we wanted a new house. So, I talked with five realtors and several lenders to write down facts. I did library research. I found pamphlets on mortgage rates and clipped articles out of every magazine I could find.

"When we found a house, two of the lenders tried to discourage us. They said we needed to save up more of a down payment. But I didn't want to wait. I knew the prices of homes would be jumping while I patiently pinched pennies. So I

talked with the builder of this new home. I said, 'I know we can do this. Please advise me on options for financing.'

She continues, "The builder said his homes were appraising for slightly more than the asking price. He pointed me to a lender who could arrange one hundred percent financing.

She continues, "We closed the deal with the savings we had. I even had a little money left to buy a few pieces of good furniture. If I hadn't approached my goal with confidence—plus the skills I'd learned in reviewing financial terminology—my husband and I would still be a good distance from home ownership."

Skills will *sustain* career goals

Because all career goals in your written plan must be supported by skills, document skills that you need to acquire. Don't assume that your skill levels will rise. Plan *how* you will obtain those skills you need. Table 10.1 can help you get started.

For example, your list might look similar to this:

I need to:

1. Take an advanced computer course
2. Learn about new hospital ER equipment
3. Take a class to gain skills in geriatric care
4. Teach a CPR course to keep sharp on instructing others

In tracking your skill levels, don't forget to write down your unique talents as part of those skills. Always rely on your special talents—for example, a willingness to do extensive research or a penchant for asking thought-provoking questions or a skill for supervising critical triage—to separate you from the crowd. You want people to remember you.

For instance, Blake, who is chief paramedic instructor at a college in New Jersey, says: "I recently hired a new instructor for our summer night school program. He is a very sensitive man who likes people. He has a talent for holding everyone's attention. I didn't want to hire someone who is boring or droll. We've had those kinds of instructors. Too many students end up dropping out. I wanted someone who was lively and inspirational. That keeps the students coming back for more."

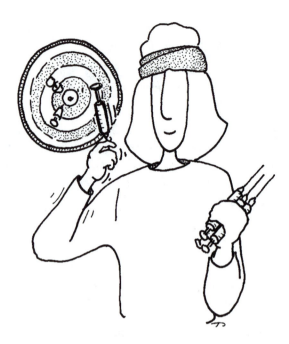

Why a written plan works

Having everything on paper is important because you won't be relying on memory for keeping track of names, dates, and people who can help you advance. Plus, if you are new in EMS, you can list the companies that are hiring and the training you need to acquire. By putting everything on paper, you can review information on a regular basis to propel yourself forward.

For example, if you've decided you would be happier in a small town, instead of Miami or Chicago, make a plan for using vacation time to visit a new locale. Do you know a friend there you might contact? What phone calls will you need to make in advance? Have you talked with your spouse? Should you check out the schools while you're there?

Your action list for moving to a new locale might include the following:

1. Talk with the EMS director of the county
2. Get a copy of my résumé to him or her
3. Call realtors in the area
4. Talk with the school board of that county
5. Tally up expenses involved in relocating

TABLE 10.1

Your career plan can be a plan you design and implement by writing up notes, lists, or charts in any fashion that makes sense to you. The following will give you an idea on how to start.

My Long-Term Goals

1. Move into management
2. Write articles on EMS
3.
4.
5.

My Short-Term Goals

1. Enroll in an accounting course
2. Find a career mentor
3.
4.
5.

My Unique Talents

1. I'm good in math
2. I stay cool under pressure
3. I'm very disciplined
4.
5.

Skills I Want to Develop

1. Better one-on-one communication
2. Helping to plan budgets
3. Writing EMS business plans
4.
5.

Good Decisions I've Already Made

1. I've moved to a good locale
2. I've upgraded my computer skills
3.
4.
5.

Obstacles I Foresee in Reaching My Goals

1. I need to polish my written English
2.
3.
4.
5.

My Strengths

1. I can organize a project well
2. I'm excellent with my patients
3. I'm good in critical triage situations
4.
5.

My Weaknesses

1. My diet is unhealthy
2. I'm impatient with my wife
3. I can't balance work and family well
4.
5.

Research I Need to Do

1. Explore jobs in management
2. Read more EMS magazines
3.
4.
5.

Goals to Which I Need to Attach a Deadline

1. Find a mentor by next month
2. Write two article queries soon
3.
4.
5.

Where I'd Like to Be at Age 80–85

1. Have a happy family life
2. Be a published author
3. I'll still serve on an EMS board
4.
5.

Although this simple list is fine for a starting point, you'll need to embellish it with more specific planning. For example, your goals for talking with certain individuals should include time frames. Don't leave details about *when* to contact people to chance. Make notes about specific dates and times to phone, fax, or e-mail. Also, you'll need to write out a list of questions to ask the EMS director, the realtor, and the school board representative.

> Ben, a county EMS director who has worked for 15 years to improve service in his area says: "Become an expert at making up lists, notes, and 'to do' action lists to achieve large goals. You have to push for what you want. If you fail, rethink or fine-tune and push again. Believe in what you want to do.
>
> "I've had people try to block my efforts. Some have said I'm power hungry and a few have tried to get me fired," he laughs. "But if your heart is in the right place, you won't pay any attention to doomsayers and saboteurs. You'll stay on your horse and ride. There will be times when you'll have to scrap a plan, redo a plan, and rely on any help you can find. But if you stick to your guns, you'll succeed."

CONSIDER YOUR FAMILY'S NEEDS

By writing down your goals and assessing how they'll impact your family, you can strategize your moves to cause the least upheaval in your personal life. In addition, planning can help you fix career problems that could be stressing your marriage and home life.

> T. J, an owner of a private ambulance company, shares how he used a written plan to end massive frustration. "My wife and I were on the verge of divorcing," he confesses. "We were so frustrated with life in general. Our income was fine, but our personal lives were a mess. I couldn't find time to visit the dentist. My wife felt like she was going insane with our packed schedule. She's always helped me with the business, but she was burning out."
>
> T. J. continues, "I sat down and listed what might help. I decided to make about 10 changes. I hired two additional part-time employees, although I couldn't really couldn't afford it. With the extra time this gave me, I took a computer course, talked with a financial planner, and attended a seminar on building a better business.
>
> "I ended up adding one substation and closing another," he explains. My personal income is actually up a little. But the real payoff of my planning is that I've found more time to be with my wife. You can work smarter, instead of harder, but you've got to make some plans for taking control of your career."

Taking the time to look at your work problems on paper helps you step outside yourself and be objective. Listing any personal problems that need to be addressed can keep your job and family from clashing, too. For example, figuring in time for your family's recreational needs is very important. Camping or other fun will balance everything out. Plans that will benefit everybody in the family are a must to work into your schedule—even if you're super busy. Figuring in recreation when you're especially busy or overloaded will keep you from burning out. Penciling in time for fun in your career plan might be its saving grace. Without time to enjoy life, you may become tempted to scrap the whole plan.

"Any time you want a career change, especially a major one, you have to talk it over with your spouse," says Jim Dernocoeur, a former paramedic in Grand Rapids, Michigan, who committed to a rigorous four-year curriculum to become a physician's assistant. "Returning to school was emotionally and physically exhausting, but absolutely worth it," he insists. "Besides," he jokes, "I knew there would come a time when I couldn't carry a 300-pound patient down a winding staircase."

Dernocoeur believes that any big career change must be a family commitment. "For the last two years of my coursework and training, I had to tell my family, 'I'm sorry, but essentially, I'm 'gone' for two years.' "

So, what if you're deeply dissatisfied, but you're scared to make a change? You might tell yourself: "I can't find financial help. I'm not smart enough to advance. I'm stuck right where I am."

Dernocoeur, who often teaches at EMS conferences on motivational and career issues, says: "You must make an overt decision to change something. I tell paramedics and prehospital personnel, 'You have specific knowledge and skills that no one else has. You're the only person stopping you.' "

In order to motivate yourself to act, consider how you might find support or resources:

- **Network continually.** Although books and articles can point you in the right direction, it is people who can give you a real boost. Talk with anyone and everyone who will share how he or she made a career climb.

    Go on-line to chat in EMS discussion groups. Or, talk with counselors at your local college who can put you in touch with other adults who are returning to school. Returning students sometimes form on-campus clubs for social and emotional support.

    Attend a career planning seminar. Go to conferences, volunteer at a hospital, or stay late after a class to ask questions of others. Your goal in networking is to discover tips for what will work to improve your situation. You don't want to make a plan that won't fly.

- **Actively scout for resources.** Locating financial help, child care, and available time are just three of the resources most people need for a significant change to become possible. Talk with a college adviser about financial aid. If you don't qualify for a grant, fill out the necessary paper-work for scholarships. Your application might impress a scholarship committee, if you promote yourself with enthusiasm.

Before you apply for a loan, find out if your local hospital will subsidize certain training for emergency responders. Or, will your employer pay for part of your schooling?

- **Take an alternative route.** For example, if child care is a problem, post a note on a college bulletin board to find a church group or parenting group who'll help. Or, approach others about forming a child care co-op, using space at a church or college.

  If personal responsibilities will interfere with future schooling, try to adjust your plan accordingly. Gill, an EMT who's studying to be a paramedic, says, "I knew I couldn't keep up my chores and yard work when I enrolled in paramedic school a few months back. So I sold my house and moved my family into an apartment. By the time I study, work, and do the clinicals required, I'm exhausted. But this is something I love. I can always buy another house."

Because the world is changing so fast, most of us know that we're past having just one career. Having to be flexible and open to new employment opportunities is a fact of life. Because employment is so unpredictable, you should make a plan for yourself to *circumvent* those plans other people will be happy to make *for you*. Besides, you will feel more in control if you fully participate in scouting for options that could benefit you. Nothing is more empowering than writing your own life story.

Although career planning sounds like a reasonable undertaking, what if you need help in visualizing your path? Maybe you don't have a great imagination. You can't picture yourself doing anything differently. You have two children, a mortgage, and a low-paying job at a rural EMS station. You feel stuck and miserable.

Try these exercises:

- **Ask yourself, "Whom do I envy?"** Write notes about people you admire. If you are impressed by someone who has achieved a certain level of success in a work role that interests you, write down the reasons you'd like to be in that type of role.
- **Plan your life backward.** Picture yourself as an 80-year-old who is saying, "I feel satisfied about the choices I've made throughout my life." Remember, you're who you are today because of the choices you made yesterday.

Professionally speaking, how much to bite off and chew, how much to demand of yourself, will become apparent when you ask, "What must I do to satisfy *me*?"

- **Let the truth set you free.** Whether you like a challenging day working EMS calls, or you eventually want to work in a more structured hospital setting, it pays to be thoroughly honest with yourself. For example, let's say that you work in a large inner-city EMS–fire division. You need to switch gears, because the truth is, you burned out three years ago. You have to force yourself to face the day.

    You've pictured yourself moving from street medic to a management position. You'd like to be involved in budget planning for your department. You'd enjoy that tremendously. Why not ask your boss if you can sit in on budget meetings? Also, find out if your division will pay for you to take one or two accounting courses.

- **Go ahead and stretch yourself.** On paper at least, why not play around with a few goals that seem out of reach. The worst that can happen is that you'll consider more alternatives. Experts say that most of us never accomplish a lot more in life than our parents did. Nobody really knows why. Could it be that we all fail to do any "stretching" exercises? We mimic what feels comfortable. In this case, it's our parents' lifestyle.

Manage your career plan by deciding to be the best at whatever you do. If you're an EMT at a small substation, polish your skills continually. Take pride in the fact that you are in public safety work—as a struggling newcomer or as a seasoned veteran. However your script unfolds, always want to do quality work. If you are just starting out in EMS, you will have the confidence to climb if you know your work is excellent.

A good example of rising through the ranks with confidence is Edgar Shilling, chief deputy of the Howard County Fire and Rescue Services in Howard County, Maryland. "I've stayed with this same department for 30 years," he explains. "I love this part of the country, so I planned all of my career moves right here—starting at the very bottom." Now, Shilling is second in command from the top, with 230 career personnel and over 200 volunteers and administrators on staff.

Shilling explains that each move in his career involved writing down plans for acquiring the training and education he would need. "Sometimes the department paid for my schooling, but many times I paid for taking seminars on personnel management or other job-related subjects," he explains. "I did career planning all along the way, and it worked for me." For a sample career plan see Table 10.2.

Having control starts and ends with planning. However, this means that decisions will have to be made, and some decisions may not be pleasant. Let your family see that you are planning for everyone's benefit. Ask for their input during the plan-

TABLE 10.2

Jim Dernocoeur, who is now a physician's assistant and an articulate speaker at EMS conferences, began his career as a paramedic. But as you will see below, Jim had a learning challenge. He didn't let that stand in his way. He offers the following advice to young paramedics and EMTs.

"My career path has been a very different type of path. I have not taken the beaten path. This is partly because I am a different type of thinker because of the unique challenges I have had to face.

"I have dyslexia, which has affected every decision I have made working toward my career goals. I was always tagged as either not very smart or not trying hard enough throughout my educational experience as a child. I was often placed in the low level performance classes. Yet, I was able to present ideas well in a verbal format."

"I developed a plan to enter the field of prehospital care. I learned what classes were needed to enter the field and what was needed to become a paramedic."

Jim's Advice to Others

1. Look at your strengths and apply them as opportunities appear.
2. Be willing to think and see things differently than others do. It means that you must be willing to make opportunities for yourself.

Jim's Career Ladder

1. I started teaching classes such as CPR and first aid classes. I became involved in teaching EMT classes.
2. I read about teaching and watched other people teach in order to improve my skills.
3. I then started helping organize EMT conferences.
4. I was given opportunities to give talks at local conferences, which lead to my presenting at national conferences.
5. I also was given an opportunity to extend my teaching skills to the written word. (With my dyslexia this was a scary and overwhelming task. With the help of my wife Kate, who has a degree in journalism, I was able to do a column. I wrote a column titled "Discussions in Paramedicine" in *JEMS*. I took the tack that I was teaching on paper. This helped me to overcome the dyslexia difficulties.)
6. I also made sure the information presented was correct, which meant that I spent a lot of time in the medical library at University of Colorado Medical School.

"This was the fulfillment of my career plan at that time and is the base from which I have built the rest of my career (as a P.A.). Many people will tell you that you cannot achieve things. Don't listen to them."

ning process. Emphasize to each family member that sacrifices may have to be made, but reassure them all that the payoffs will be worth it to the family as a whole.

Keeping track of the progress you are making, the progress you are *not* making, and the options you might need to try all go into career planning. By fine-tuning your strategies, noting what you need to do differently, and outlining small steps to take *when nothing seems to be working* is what will make your plan fly. Keep thinking of doors to knock on, letters to write, and ideas to research that are different from what you have already tried.

Whether you need more personal satisfaction, more of a challenge, or more economic security, your plan can be your ticket. When you're 80, you can truthfully say, "I feel good about the choices I've made. I did what it took to satisfy me."

In order to write a better career plan:

- **Make a list of the activities you have enjoyed during the past few years.** Evaluate why you enjoy participating in these activities.
- **Write down all of the skills you possess.** Include "people skills," good communication skills, decision-making skills, and problem-solving skills, along with your medical expertise.
- **Write down two or three career choices.** Pencil in the benefits of each choice into your plan.
- **Make a list of professional journals, magazines, and newsletters you need to read.** Write down where you could obtain older copies or borrow new ones.
- **Develop and maintain a professional portfolio.** Document your work and related accomplishments in it. It's easy to forget what you fail to write. Keep track of your accomplishments on an ongoing basis by keeping a notebook with you at all times.

HOW TO WRITE A BETTER LIFE PLAN

In creating a plan to improve the quality of your personal life and close relationships, remember to pencil in changes for taking better care of yourself. It is easier to nurture others when you nurture yourself. Without a plan for taking care of youself, there will be an emptiness to your life. Putting off doing things for yourself might work for a short time, but this kind of neglect will catch up with you.

In dealing with your spouse and children, try to talk very openly about your needs. Make it clear to them why you pencil in time for extra sleep or time to run before dinner. However, *never* make your family feel that your needs are more important than theirs. Always ask about the needs and concerns of those close to you.

Inquire about their stress levels. Be concerned about their personal needs, even if you can't readily assist in meeting those needs.

> "I used to give my family long lectures about my stress," says Evan, an EMT. "I'd beg off on doing this or that, so I could stay home and unwind. My teenage son pointed me in a better direction one day. He said, 'Dad, if you think running calls is tough, you ought to try passing Algebra II.' Well, I had to laugh out loud. He was just saying, 'Give me a break here. You're not the only person with stress.'"

> Evan continues, "I started focusing on ways to dump my stress faster. I bought a mountain bike so I could join my son for rides in the afternoon. I started taping biographies off cable TV to watch later with my wife. I had to diligently plan how to interrupt my old coping mechanisms. I've had to work at redirecting my energies.

> "I used to sit in my recliner, sip a mixed drink, and mentally rehearse tragedies I'd experienced all day. But this wasn't helping anyone—myself included. The mountain biking has been great for me. I'm hoping that eventually my wife and daughter will take up mountain biking, too. That would be ideal for us as a family."

Families who experience more closeness are those who enjoy planning activities together. If your budget won't permit a costly vacation, plan one-day trips close to home. If you can't afford to take everyone out to dinner every weekend, plan inexpensive cookouts or friendly card games. Write these activities into your daily planner, and make family closeness a priority in your general life plan. When your children are grown, they will remember the effort and time you invested to be with them. Without planning, you will not as likely find as much time for family togetherness.

Jay Fitch, Ph.D., president of an EMS consulting firm who was introduced in Chapter 7, believes that prehospital care providers can often use the flexibility of their jobs to do special things for their families. "For instance, EMTs can drop by their child's school for lunch on certain days, while some parents in other jobs can't manage this," he says. "You've got to be innovative to make it all work." Table 10.3 is an example of a long-term plan.

Make all of your plans with your family or friends very doable. Instead of making elaborate plans, do everything you can to simplify your life. Don't believe that doing more is always the better route. Simple solutions to problems will leave you and others in your life feeling more in control.

> "I used to think about moving my family to a bigger house," says Martin, who's worked as an EMT for 20 years while running a small family-owned store in his community. "We'd reached a point where our possessions were overflowing. We were very crowded, but I didn't want a bigger mortgage.

TABLE 10.3

Mike Grill, a firefighter–paramedic of the Sierra Vista Fire Department in Arizona, works closely with co-author Jeff Dyar in an EMS consulting company, The Far View Group.

Mike also teaches at the National Fire Academy in Emmitsburg, Maryland. Below, he shares his personal 5-year plan and his 10-year vision:

Michael Thomas Grill's Personal Goals Written in January 1999

At the End of Five Years

1. I will have achieved geographical independence; I can live anywhere I desire and still have a quality life.
2. The Far View Group, of which I am a key stakeholder, will be a recognized leader in providing consulting services to all EMS-related organizations.
3. I will be speaking at least 12 times a year.
4. I will be in outstanding physical and mental health.
5. My relationship with my family (Lacey, Sam, and Moe) will still be one of fulfillment, joy, and love.

My 10-year vision:

I will be an internationally recognized public speaker on establishing quality-driven fire departments and EMS agencies. To do this, I will become a nationally recognized leader in the United States Fire Service through constant and never-ending improvement.

Deadline: 2005

Step 1: I will continue my education through the CPM Program, and then I will work on a master's degree; while doing this, I will continue to write, speak, and teach at The National Fire Academy.

Step 2: After 3 to 5 years' experience at the supervisory level with the Sierra Vista Fire Department, I will become a fire chief or a chief officer of a fire department. I'll continue with step 1 during this process.

Step 3: Apply what I've learned in my new chief officer's position. Also, I will gain the experience that will lend credibility to what I speak about in an international forum of fire service–EMS leaders. I'll continue with Step 1 during this process.

"I solicited my family's help in tossing and cleaning out what we didn't need. We streamlined everything. We donated tons of items to charity. Before long, our house looked more livable. We're still here and we're very happy. The children were relieved they didn't have to leave the neighborhood. A lifestyle jam-packed with material possessions can be the source of a lot of stress. By simplifying, you're saying, 'I don't want my possessions to own me.' It takes a plan to de-junk your life."

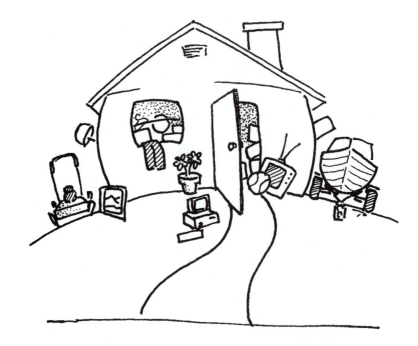

Finding your way around obstacles, either in your personal life or in your career, is important to controlling stress. By feeling blocked, you're going to feel frustrated and defeated. In order to pave the way to your goals, try to target what's getting in the way of progress. For example, are you failing to work on your marriage? Do you just keeping hoping things will change? Or, is your spouse's attitude preventing you from returning to paramedic school? Would your spouse be more committed to helping you return to school if you could support new career decisions for him or her?

By writing down all areas of your life that need attention, you'll figure out which areas to address first. By prioritizing, you can manage to change those things you need to change. Naturally, you want to create the best career you can. But also, through planning, you can figure out how to enjoy your career. You can figure out how to have more control over your work life and your personal life.

Stretching yourself to grow and develop might not be easy. But when you became an emergency responder, you became part of a special calling. You decided to be on the front lines of life. When others are at risk, in deep trouble, or totally unable to help themselves, you want to play a role in reestablishing their safety. You help to honor this calling when you take good care of yourself. Keeping yourself safe both emotionally and physically will ensure that others can depend on you.

Constantly strive to deal with your stress *before it gets out of hand.* Find out what's possible to do and learn to let go of what you can't change. Never try to control everything, but do try to find meaning and purpose in all of your experiences. Keep looking for choices in life. Take a few risks. Always include the risk of reaching out to other people. Never stop needing contact and closeness with people.

In order to lower your stress, you do have to protect yourself emotionally in lots of ways. But always strive to heal quickly when someone or something has hurt you. Never stay down for long. Keep your spirit alive by having a love affair with life. Focus on where you want to go. Don't get caught up in counting the steps to getting there. Focus on taking the steps.

Balance does not come from one event. Balance comes from how you live every single day. The small control buttons and the small choices do add up. They give you power over every situation. As you actively use the power you have each moment, you will feel more balance. You will feel in control of managing your stress. Look for the options, look for the choices, and monitor what's happening to you. With enough good changes, you will improve the quality of your life.

REVIEW ACTIVITIES

1. Name one important goal you would like to reach within 12 months. Break the goal down into steps. Plan an action to-do list to ensure the completion of your goal. Do you foresee any obstacles to reaching your goal? How could you realistically remove those obstacles?

2. Why will planning your most important goals on paper help you to evaluate your progress?

3. List your top 10 professional skills. Name 5 more you would like to add in the near future.

4. What unique talent separates you from others? How might this talent help you to market yourself, should you become unemployed?

5. Why is it important to validate the needs of your family members?

6. Name two personal goals you'd like to accomplish with a family member or friend. State why these goals are important to you.

7. List three small improvements you could pencil into your self-care plan this week. What benefits would you gain if you kept doing them for six months?

8. Name three professional people you should network with in the future. How could you make a plan to introduce yourself to these people? Why would their expertise help you?

9. What would be the ultimate career goal for you? If you were 80 years old and looking back over your life, how would it make you feel to have obtained this?

FOR SUPERVISORS

1. One of your employees has come to you for advice. This person needs productive feedback concerning his or her job performance over the past year. Would you be open and honest with this individual, or would you tend to avoid being too critical? How could failure to assess this person's weakness hurt him or her? How could you sandwich your criticisms between two thick layers of praise in order to protect this person's ego?

2. Let's say that your job has recently pulled your focus away from your family. You realize it is time to regain your overall life balance. How could you begin to offer more of yourself to your family? Name one way you could adjust your schedule to allow two additional hours per week for family time.

CLASS PROJECT

1. Have several class members describe how they overcame personal difficulties or roadblocks to achieve success. Have the class vote on their favorite story. Ask each participant to share with the class his or her best advice on how to motivate oneself.

APPENDIX

SUGGESTED READING LIST:

Life Strategies: Doing What Works/Doing What Matters
By Phillip C. McGraw, PhD
Hyperion/New York 1990

Codependent No More
Melody Beattie
(Harper Collins) 1987

If You Haven't Got Time To Do It Right When Will You
    Have Time To Do It Over?
By Jeffrey J. Mayer
Simon & Schuster 1990

The Time Trap
By Alec Mackenzie
AMACOM 1997

The Complete Idiot's Guide To Managing Stress
By Jeff Davidson, MBA, CMC
Alpha Books/New York 1997

Give And Take: The Secret To Marital Compatibility
By Williard F. Harley, Jr.
Fleming H. Revell (Baker Book House
    Company/Michigan) 1996

Love Busters: Overcoming Habits That Destroy
    Romantic Love
By Williard F. Harley, Jr., Ph.D.
Fleming H. Revell Company/New York 1992

Touche Ross Guide to Personal Financial Management
By John R. Connell
LaVerne L. Dotson
W. Thomas Porter
Robert E. Zobel
Prentice-Hall/New York 1987

First Things First
By Stephen R. Covey
Roger Merrill
Rebecca R. Merrill
Simon & Schuster/New York 1995

Success Is A Choice
By Rick Pitino with Bill Reynolds
Broadway Books/New York 1997

Daily Marriage Builders for Couples
By Fred & Florence Littauer
World Publishing/Nashville 1997

The Leader in You
Dale Carnegie & Associates
Pocket Books New York 1993

Managing Would Be Easy . . . If It Weren't For the
    People
By Patricia J. Addresso, PhD
AMACOM/New York 1996

What Color Is Your Parachute?
By Richard Nelson Bolles
Ten Speed Press/California 1999

What To Say When You Talk To Yourself
By Shad Helmstetter, PhD
Pocket Books/New York 1982

Your Personal NetMoney
(A Guide to the Personal Finance Revolution on the
    Internet)
Edited by Michael Wolff
Dell/New York 1997

INTERNET WEBSITES:

Stress related sites: coped exactly for accuracy:

http://www.scl.ncal.kaiperm.org/healthinfo/stress/
    index.html
(Kaiser Permanente's Reference: Stress page)

http://www.teachhealth.com/
Medical Basis of Stress page

www.virtualpsych.com/stress/fancyindex.htm
Virtual psych page

career sites:

http://www.careerlab.com/art_25hottips.htm
Careerlab page

http://www.bgsu.edu/offices/careers/process/process.html
Career Planning Process Page:

http://www.careercity.com/
(Career City page)

frugal living sites

http://www.sirius.com/~lindah/frugal/
(Frugal Family Living page)

http://pages.prodigy.com/frugal_tightwad/index.htm
(Tightwad page)

http://cheetah.spots.ab.ca/~ics/home.html
(Best Links and Tips)

http://www.covco.com/nannie/frugal.html
(My Frugal Page)

INDEX

To purchase additional copies of

BURNOUT TO BALANCE: EMS Stress
Hopson/Hopson/Dyar

0-13-007806-9

have your credit card information ready and call

1-800-282-0693

or fax

515-284-6719

You can also mail your order to

Centrobe Order Processing Center
PO Box 11071
Des Moines, IA 50336

To purchase additional copies of

BURNOUT TO BALANCE: EMS Stress
Hopson/Hopson/Dyar

0-13-007806-9

have your credit card information ready and call

1-800-282-0693

or fax

515-284-6719

You can also mail your order to

Centrobe Order Processing Center
PO Box 11071
Des Moines, IA 50336